Fisheries Information System for India

Fisheries Information System for India

Author

Dr. M Jayapradeep

Foreword by

Dr. R Raman Nair

SATISH SERIAL PUBLISHING HOUSE
403, Express Tower, Commercial Complex
Azadpur, Delhi-110033 (India)
Phone : 011-27672852, Fax : 91-11-27672046
e-mail : info@satishserial.com, hkjain1975@yahoo.com
Website : www.satishserial.com

Published by :

SATISH SERIAL PUBLISHING HOUSE
403, Express Tower, Commercial Complex, Azadpur, Delhi-110033 (INDIA)
Phone : 011-27672852 Fax : 91-11-27672046
E-mail : info@satishserial.com, hkjain1975@yahoo.com

ISBN 978-93-86200-22-8

Composed, Designed & Printed in India

About the Author

Dr. M Jayapradeep has MA in Political Science, MLISc and MPhil in Library and Information Science. Awarded PhD for his work on Fisheries Informatics from Karpagam University in 2014. Served Indian Air Force, Biotechnology Information Centre (Government of India), Kerala Agricultural University, Kerala University of Fisheries and Ocean Studies, and is presently Librarian, SVN College of Engineering, Mavelikkara, Kerala. Has long experience in guiding research students and teachers. Areas of interests are informatics and knowledge management. Published/presented numerous research papers in journals/conferences. Editorial board member of national and international journals in LIS. Advisory of the 'Informatics Studies' an International Scholarly Journal.

Dedicated to

The LIS teachers who graced the
'distance learners'
invisibly in the realm of
'Distance Education Programmes'

Foreword

Fisheries sector is considered as one of the important productive and developmental sectors. About 3 per cent of the India's economy is attributed to Fisheries. Various institutions have sprang-up in fisheries sector for knowledge generation. The information or knowledge thus generated has to be applied in education, research, development through context based timely dissemination or extension in a speedy, effective and efficient manner for the sustainable development of the sector. But it is observed that there are various constraints in the information cycle from the generation, production, dissemination and access to its effective use and sharing in fisheries sector. It necessitates serious efforts involving library and information systems to provide timely and reliable information to support decision making, policy formulation, and sustainable development in fisheries sector.

The present work of Sri M Jayapradeep is the result of a comprehensive study on fisheries information resources and services in India with the intention to evolve and implement a national level Fisheries Information Management System that can help to restructure education, redefine scientific research and reorganize the media of communication to an inter-active and de-centralised mode. The study proposes practical suggestions and solutions for better integration of information into the main stream of fisheries sector. It measures and analyses the present status of information system and services in Indian fisheries sector. Mixed methodologies and instruments for data collection have been adopted by the author who has treated the problems in a holistic way. The samples used consist of institutions and stakeholders in the sub-systems of education, planning, development, research, extension, trading and communities in the fisheries sector. The study considers various indicators to represent the nature and extent of the research problem. The research report is suitably paraphrased for book and the observations and solutions are given in respective chapters as conclusions.

The author recommends for institutionalizing the fisheries information sector and provides a detailed plan for the same by elaborating its organization, design and components. The contents are illuminative, the observations are fairly mature and the analysis of the issues has been critical throughout. It also goes beyond discussing the mere transactional and instrumental quality of the fisheries information services to a more caring and humane system. The responsibility of Library and Information System (LIS) profession in reaching the un-reached and in transmitting the strength of knowledge to the grass roots' level that shall garner sense of credibility to the LIS profession is also discussed in the work.

Several market places that collectively address the information needs of the end user are (1) integrated library systems (2) online databases (3) web based resources (4) digital library collections and (5) e-books and e-journals. The enabling technology is the network centric client-server environment and the enabling software is TCP/IP. These aspects have been taken care of in a substantial way, serving the book for general reading as well as an information source for decision makers, LIS professionals, researchers and students of fisheries as well as library science. The conceptual framework and research methods are given in detail so as to serve as a reference guide for the LIS researchers. I am very happy to recommend this book to the researchers and scholars in the field of Fisheries Informatics in India. The suggestions contained in the book may provide useful clues to the policy makers and planners engaged in informatics.

Thiruvananthapuram **R. Raman Nair**

[Dr. R. Raman Nair was educated at University of Kerala and Banaras Hindu University. He has associated with major digitization projects including Web Archives of Kerala Legislative Assembly Proceedings, and Mahatma Gandhi University Open Access Ph D Theses Digital Library. He was a member of the National Committee on Submission and Access to Electronic Theses and Dissertations in Universities in India which envisioned Shodganga and concerned clauses in Ph D Regulation of UGC to bring doctoral dissertations of the Indian universities to public domain. Has served as University Librarian of Kerala Agricultural University and Mahatma Gandhi University (MGU) and as Officer on Special Duty (Library) of Central University of Kerala where he developed a Knowledge Base on International Studies (IS Knowledge Base). He has envisioned and initiated the establishment of Centre for Advanced Research in Library and Information Science at MGU. Organized many national and international training programmes on ICT under Ministries of Science and Technology, Agriculture and other agencies of Government of India, got the SM Ganguly National Award in 1998 and has numerous published books on Information Science and related subjects].

Preface

Information is an ingredient, a problem-solving tool and a key factor for transformation of the society. Fisheries sector that occupies a crucial place in the socio-economic development of the country needs information in various formats by all the stakeholders from policy makers to the grass root level fishers and fish farmers for the sustainable development of the sector. Nevertheless it is observed that the fisheries information sector is a neglected area in terms of knowledge generation, policy formulations, programmes, studies, research, services, systems and institutionalization.

The book consolidates fragmented approaches taken at several levels at the Centre and the States that need to be coordinated, integrated and harmonized into a coherent whole of Information Management System that is based on cooperation, resource sharing and up-to-date scalable technology. The book addresses the issues of fisheries information and knowledge systems in India, and suggests methods for equal opportunity for access of fisheries information by all the stakeholders for the optimum utilization of information and knowledge in fisheries sector.

The study is presented in 10 chapters. Chapter 1 gives a brief outline of the research problem and the study. Chapter 2 makes general review of the classical, neoclassical and current literature relating to the subject. Chapter 3 presents the conceptual framework and methodology followed in this study. Chapter 4 gives an account of the fisheries sector of India, pertinently noting the decisive role of information and knowledge for the sustainable development of the Indian fisheries sector. Chapter 5 furnishes a detailed account of the institutions, revealing the information capacity of the sector. Chapter 6 makes a detailed account of fisheries information sector in the State of Kerala. Chapter 7 forms the analysis of the fisheries information capacity of the sector and patron views of information resources and services in the sector. Chapter 8 maps fisheries informatics and communication and Chapter 9 form the case for implementation of the Fisheries Information System of India (FISI). Chapter 10 put forth the agenda for national planning of Fisheries Information Management.

I have tried to unravel the different aspects of fisheries information with new interpretations to draw attention of all concerned and also to attract their expert opinion. I admit that the shortcomings of this work are wholly due to my inadvertence.

This book is the result of the research undertaken for award of Ph D at Karpagam University, Coimbatore. It would not have been possible without the kind assistance received from several persons and institutions throughout length and breadth of India, various Central and State Government Departments, Directors of National research institutions, Deans of Fisheries Colleges, NGO workers, fishermen, fish farmers and other stakeholders of fisheries sector. I wish to record my indebtedness to them all. I am also indebted to the scientists, teachers, students, librarians from fisheries sector, fishers and fish farmers for their cooperation and responses to the questionnaires. I gratefully acknowledge the Study Grant provided by the Indian Council of Social Science Research, Southern Regional Centre, Hyderabad for my research work.

I express my deep sense of gratitude to Dr R Raman Nair, former University Librarian of Kerala Agricultural University and Mahatma Gandhi University. His expertise, support, guidance and encouragement helped me to complete the work in time and to publish it as a book. I am also indebted to him for writing foreword to this book. I also thank Dr S Ally Sornam, Head, Dept of Library and Information Science, and Dean, Research and Development, Bishop Heber Autonomous University, Trichy whose suggestions helped me immensely to improve the work. I owe to my wife Prema and, my son Jayasankar for completing the research work.

The courage and strength to endure hardships during my studies and to paraphrase the work to publish as a book came from my faith in the ever gracious, all embracing Eternal Mother. I remember Her lotus feet in all humility.

I respectfully bow before the lotus feet of my Guru, Srimad Hariswamikal, Acharya of the Age. I fondly hope that this humble work which I could undertake due to Mother's and Guru's Divine Grace will be of use to the future researchers, students and professionals.

I express my gratitude and indebtedness to all the celebrated scholars whose works have been quoted in this book.

My deep appreciation and thanks to Satish Serial Publishing House, Delhi for the commendable work of organizing the publication of this book with rapt care and bringing out with its fineness.

M Jayapradeep

Abbreviations

AC	:	Accredited Colleges
AAU	:	Assam Agricultural Univesity
ASFA	:	Aquatic Science and Fisheries Abstracts
BCE	:	Before Common Era
BSKKV	:	Dr. Balasaheb Sawant Konkan Krishi Vidypeeth
CAU	:	Central Agricultural University
CASABF	:	Centre of Advanced Study in Aquatic Biology and Fisheries
CASMB	:	Centre of Advanced Study in Marine Biology
CE	:	Common Era
CeRA	:	Consortium for e-Resources in Agriculture
CIBA	:	Central Institute of Brackishwater Aquaculture
CICEF	:	Central Institute of Coastal Engineering for Fishery
CIFA	:	Central Institute of Freshwater Aquaculture
CIFE	:	Central Institute of Fisheries Education
CIFI	:	Central Institute of Fisheries Informatics
CIFNET	:	Central Institute of Fisheries Nautical and Engineering Training
CIFRI	:	Central Inland Capture Fisheries Research Institute
CIFT	:	Central Institute of Fisheries Technology
CL	:	Central Library
CMFRI	:	Central Marine Fisheries Research Institute
CMLRE	:	Centre for Marine Living Resources and Ecology
CNREP	:	Centre for Natural Resource, Economics and Policy
CoF	:	College of Fisheries
CoFSc	:	College of Fisheries Science
CSIR	:	Council of Scientific & Industrial Research
CU SFC	:	Calicut University Self Financing College
CUSAT	:	Cochin University of Science and Technology
DA	:	Digital Archives

DAHDF	:	Department of Animal Husbandry, Dairying and Fisheries
DCFR	:	Directorate of Coldwater Fisheries Research
DF& Agnc	:	Dept. of Fisheries and other Agencies under the Department
DKMA	:	Directorate of Knowledge Management in Agriculture
DoF	:	Department of Fisheries
DST	:	Department of Science and Technology
e-Book	:	Electronic Book
EIS	:	Electronic Information Source
e-Journal	:	Electronic Journal
ETD	:	Electronic Theses & Dissertations
FAO	:	Food and Agriculture Organization of the United Nations
FCRI	:	Fisheries College and Research Institute
FISHCOPFED	:	National Federation of Fishermen's Cooperatives Ltd
FISI	:	Fisheries Information System of India
FISNet	:	Fisheries Information System Network
FS Pyp	:	Fisheries Research Station, Puthuvypu
FSI	:	Fishery Survey of India
GADVASU	:	Guru Angad Dev Veterinary and Animal Sciences University
GBPUAT	:	GB Pant University of Agriculture & Technology
GDP	:	Gross Domestic Product
GIS	:	Geographical Information System
IAMSLIC	:	The International Association of Aquaculture and Marine Science Libraries and Information Centres
ICAR	:	Indian Council of Agricultural Research
ICES	:	International Council for the Exploration of the Sea
ICSF	:	International Collective in Support of Fishworkers
ICT	:	Information and Communication Technology
IFT	:	Institute of Fisheries Technology
IGKVV	:	Indira Gandhi KrishiVishwa Vidyalaya

INCOIS	:	Indian National Centre for Ocean Information System
INFLIBNET	:	Information and Library Network of UGC
ISO	:	International Organization for Standardization
IT	:	Information Technology
JAU	:	Junagadh Agricultural University
JSTOR	:	Journal Storage
KAU	:	Kerala Agricultural University
KGEU	:	Knowledge Generation, Exchange and Utilization
KM	:	Knowledge Management
KU	:	Kerala University
KUFOS	:	Kerala University of Fisheries and Ocean Studies
Kum	:	Kumarakom
KVAFSU	:	Karnataka Veterinary Animal & Fisheries Science University
KVK	:	Krishi Vigyan Kendra
LAN	:	Local Area Network
LIS	:	Library and Information Science
MAFSU	:	Maharashtra Animal and Fisheries Science University
MARC	:	MAchine-Readable Cataloging
Matsya	:	Matsyafed
Matsyafed	:	Kerala State Cooperative Federation for Fisheries Development Limited
MG	:	MG University
MoES	:	Ministry of Environment and Forest
MPEDA	:	Marine Products Export Development Authority
MPUAT	:	Maharana Pratap University of Agriculture & Technology
MSSRF	:	MS Swaminathan Research Foundation
NBFGR	:	National Bureau of Fish Genetic Resources
NCAER	:	National Council of Applied Economic Research
NDUAT	:	Narendra Deva University of Agriculture and Technology
NFDB	:	National Fisheries Development Board

NIFAM	:	National Institute of Fisheries Administration and Management
NIFPHATT	:	National Institute of Fisheries Post Harvest Technology and Training
NIO	:	National Institute of Oceanography
NIO-K	:	NIO Kochi
NIRD	:	National Institute of Rural Development & Panchayti Raj
NISO	:	National Information Standards Organization
NKN	:	National Knowledge Network
OCLC	:	Online Computer Library Center, Inc
OPAC	:	Online Public Access Catalogue
OUAT	:	Odisha University of Agriculture and Technology
R&D	:	Research and Development
RC	:	Regional Centre
SAU	:	State Agricultural University
SDI	:	Selective Dissemination of Information
SKUAST-K	:	Sher-e-Kashmir University of Agricultural Science and Technology-Kashmir
SMS	:	School of Marine Science
SVUT	:	Sri Venkateswara Veterinary University
SWAN	:	State Wide Area Network
TNFU	:	Tamil Nadu Fisheries University
UGC	:	University Grants Commission
UNESCO	:	UN Educational, Scientific & Cultural Organization
UNISIST	:	UN International Scientific Information System
URL	:	Uniform Resource Locator
UT	:	Union Territory
VIC	:	Village Information Centre
VKC	:	Village Knowledge Centre
VRC	:	Village Resource Centre
WBUAFS	:	West Bengal University of Animal and Fishery Science
ZSI	:	Zoological Survey of India

List of Tables

List of Figures

Contents

Chapter-1

Introduction

Fishing is one of the oldest recorded sources of livelihood in India. Fishery sector occupies an important place in the socio-economic development of the country. It is a source of livelihood to about 15 million people engaged fully, partially or in subsidiary activities, with an equally impressive segment of the population engaged in ancillary activities associated with fisheries and aquaculture. Indian fisheries industry includes culture, capture, post-harvest handling, marketing and processing of fish and fisheries products.

Indian fisheries and aquaculture sector has been recognized as the fastest growing food production system during the last three decades. Its contribution towards national economies, livelihood, food and nutritional security, employment generation and foreign exchange earnings have been enormous. It is certain that the sector will be playing a prominent role of a revenue earner and food supplier for the nation due to the growing demand for food and with constraints on the land availability for the agriculture. This is contingent upon sustainable development of the sector.

Technological transformation that can boost fisheries production consists of improvements in material inputs, farming techniques, storage technology, research, education and extension. Effective integration of these factors relates to the adequate information flow. Fisheries research conducted at various research institutions under Union and State Governments at huge public expense generate new technologies. National Agricultural Research System of India, one of the largest of its kind in the world is engaged in production and dissemination of agricultural information including fisheries. The feed companies, seed companies, certification agencies, water resource development agencies, planning and administration agencies, market and price commissions, export agencies, development boards, Non-governmental Organisations (NGOs) and many other agencies are also involved in production of information relevant to fisheries sector. But, fisheries information is not easily available from any system, be it *Matsya Bhavans* in the villages or specialized institutions and agencies such as ICAR. The current scenario is far from satisfactory in spite of resources and e-infrastructure developed in the sector by using enormous public fund.

India is evolving into a developed economy and a more equitable society where in knowledge and entrepreneurship are decisive factors. Information management acts as a forerunner for the development of the society. Therefore, fisheries being an important sector involved in food production, evaluation of existing information resources and services of the sector has become very essential for assessing the status and revamping the information scenario of the sector.

Several functionaries at various levels of the government and other organizations are involved in decision-making, planning, research, development, education and extension in fisheries sector of India. Timely availability of quality information is *sine qua non* in this vital economic and food sector. The development and effective management of fisheries is generally the result of the quality information, research and statistics generated in the sector. Vis-à-vis, information services develop in response to the stakeholders' needs and activities. Nevertheless, there are various constraints in the cycle from the generation to utilization in the sector, which provide ample scope for detailed studies on fisheries information resources and services to mitigate the issues relating to access, sharing, distribution and utilization of fisheries information.

Need for the Study

There are numerous institutions of the Central and the State Governments for teaching, learning, research, extension and development in fisheries sector. The capital and recurring investment met for them are substantial. If they are to fulfill their objectives, they require quality information support. Presently, a comprehensive information base for the sector is not established. Fisheries information bases are dispersed over numerous institutions and organizations spread throughout the country. Proper access to information and its utilization is a problem. The sector has not addressed the right of the primary stakeholders for fisheries information and services for their vocation and profit making on equal terms with that of the other stakeholders. These factors necessitates a detailed study so that the principles that can serve as starting point for design, operation and functioning of an information management system for the sector could be drawn.

Objectives

Systematic investigation and evaluation of the information resources, facilities and services of the organizations engaged in fisheries education, research, extension and development in India as a whole and Kerala in particular. This study evaluates information resources and services in fisheries sector in India by assessing the current scenario of information availability to stakeholders and to determine the factors that affect efficiency and extension of information services in the fisheries sector. This study has the additional objectives of offering certain suggestions for information management in fisheries sector by proposing a plan for establishing a fisheries information system and network for India.

Hypothesis

The major hypotheses of this study are that the Fisheries Sector holds relevant and valuable information resources but stakeholders lacks access to them and the sector lacks proper information resource management and resource sharing programmes for the provisions of information services and the effective utilization of available information resources. It is also hypothesized that the sector needs a fisheries information system for improving information flow in the sector.

Methodology

Summary of methods and instruments of the study is presented in Table 1. Detailed account of methodology of the study is given in Chapter 3.

Table 1. Research Methods and Instruments of the Study

Methods	Survey, Interview, Field Visits, Observation
Respondents	Library and Information Professionals, Officials, Peoples' Representatives, Managers, Scientists, Teachers, Activists, Students, Fishers, Farmers, Traders
Population	Stakeholders those who use information and those who need information in fisheries sector for their vocations and profit making
Instrument	Questionnaires 1 to 5
Mode	E-mail, Post, Visits to Home/Office/Institution/Village
Sample Selection	Stratified, Quota, Random, Judgment and Observation

Scope and Limitations of the Study

Comprehensive study of the status of fisheries information resources, services and systems in India is essential to evolve and develop an Information Management System. Such a system can support to restructure education, redefine scientific research and reorganize the media of communication to an inter-active and decentralized mode. The scope of the study is broad. Nevertheless, it is also an advantage as it looks at the different dimensions and offers a better understanding of the problem in a holistic manner. As a piecemeal approach may not yield valid and useful result, a broad sweep study is undertaken to arrive at viable solutions to the problems in fisheries information sector.

Significance of the Study

Resources, services, systems, frameworks and policies for fisheries information in India are fragmented. This lacuna leads to limited coordination and ineffectual strategies in the sector. The present study attempts to suggest proper solutions for information management covering resource sharing, networking and deliverance of information services to the stakeholders effectively and efficiently with a futuristic view of Knowledge Management Systems in fisheries sector. India being a signatory to the international agreements for sustainable fisheries development, it is very important to strengthen the information system with physical, economical, technical and human resources under the new regime.

❑❑❑

Chapter-2

Research on Fisheries Information Management

Libraries serving specific category of users especially on specialized subjects became common only in the second quarter of the twentieth century. In India, the first initiative to study agricultural library system was carried out in 1957. It was the Report of the Shaw and Rao Committee constituted by ICAR on Library and Bibliographical Services for Agricultural Teaching and Research in India (Raman Nair 2004). Fisheries, though a sub-set of agriculture, is an emerging sector now. For the present study, the results of literature search on broader terms of 'fisheries information resources, services and systems' and search in Bibliographic databases such as CABI (CAB International) Abstracts, LISA (Library and Information Science Abstracts), and the useful Web sources are consulted. Considering the dramatic developments taken place in information transfer and literature output on ICT during the past two decades, the research done after the year 2000 are reviewed. Some studies with far reaching effects are exceptions. Review of Literature for the study revealed that research studies related to fisheries libraries, information resources, services and systems are only very few.

Neo Classic Literature

Johnson (1986) identified the gap between the need and the supply of information, essential services required in marine sector and gave a design of Marine Fisheries Information System, linking all the 15 Regional and Field Centres of CMFRI with the headquarters at Kochi as apex database of Marine Information. Subbaiah (1985) in his Ph D thesis on 'Conceptual framework for an Indian National Agricultural Information System (INAGRIS)' gave a conceptual framework for implementing national level Agricultural Information System.

Sujatha (2007) investigated the factors affecting the use of Electronic Information Sources (EIS) in the fisheries colleges and research institutes in South India. The study suggested strategies to improve EIS use and services by libraries such as imparting training to users and staff, resource sharing and collaboration. The frequency of use of EIS, characteristics of the respondents, fisheries education in South India, infrastructure, etc were the areas covered in the study. Raman Nair (2004) in his study on factors affecting quality of agricultural and farm information services in Kerala stressed the need for an efficient information system for agricultural education, research, extension and development. The study brought out lacuna in the library and information systems in agriculture sector which includes fisheries. The study proposed steps to ensure accessibility to full agricultural information available from worldwide sources to the institutions and users in the State.

Jayapradeep and Raman Nair (2012A) evaluated the information capacity of the aquatic and fisheries institutions in the region of Cochin, Kerala numbering 29 within the geographical proximity of 6 km radius that is in an advantageous position for information resource sharing and cooperative information services. The study suggested that the national fisheries institutions under ICAR in Cochin could play the central role in the regional information network activities in the field of aquatic and fisheries sector.

Jayapradeep and Raman Nair in an another study (2012B) advocated the need for holistic view and initiative for implementation of Knowledge Management (KM) in fisheries sector through cooperation among SAARC (South Asian Association for Regional Cooperation) member States. The study opined that KM could mutually benefit the members by exchange of scientific and technological information for the success of the regional projects on Food Safety and Bio-security initiatives including containment of Trans-boundary Fish diseases and also help deriving overall national economic growth and welfare of the people. The study emphasized the role of LIS professionals and the need for reinventing professional concepts in knowledge-based environment and KM systems. The study suggested a fisheries portal on the lines of Pacific Islands Marine Resources Information System (PIMRIS) for SAARC regional cooperation.

Sujatha and Mudhol (2009) evaluated electronic information services in four fisheries college libraries in South India and identified the challenges in providing these services and emphasized the need of strengthening institutional capacity for access to fisheries information. In another study, Sujatha and Mudhol (2006) identified some of the important national and international electronic databases in fisheries and aquaculture research and management.

Raman Nair (2007) evaluated the resources, facilities and services of information units of fisheries related organizations and gave suggestions for establishing an information system and network for maximum utilization of the information resources in the wake of the emerging world's trade regime. Sujatha, Mudhol and Murthy (2006) examined the need for establishing National Fisheries Information System, with a central role assigned to ICAR. Ibeun (2004) examined the situation in Nigeria regarding information networking in fisheries and aquaculture sciences and its future prospects. He proposed a National Fisheries Information Network to enhance resource sharing within the country.

FAO (2004) Fisheries Report No. 740 reviewed the Fisheries library networking activities as a basis for planning future collaboration to improve access to fisheries information and to promote information resources sharing in African countries. The Workshop suggested dissemination of fisheries publications, full-text online fisheries journals, open source software, network focal points, the use of standard methodologies, etc., to enhance information exchange and technology for document delivery.

Kadzamira, Ngwira and Salanje (2003) proposed mechanisms for the sharing of information resources and improved access to inland fisheries and aquaculture information and documentation in Malawi, a developing African country. The study pointed out that the fisheries libraries were not satisfying the information needs of users due to the inadequate information resources and lack of trained library personnel. They suggested a national focal point for coordination, resource sharing, training and adoption of technologies for improved access to the information. The bibliometric studies by Jayasree and Subbiah (2000) had brought out many facets on India's contribution to the world literature of fisheries and aquaculture. Citation impact, choice of journals by scientists, ranking of institutions and places, contributions of different institutions, etc., have been brought out by the study. The need for standard formats and interoperability of databases are stressed by the study after noting disparities rampant in one and the same database.

FAO Literature

FAO has brought out many publications dealing with networking and resources sharing in fisheries especially with regard to African countries. Code of Conduct for Responsible Fisheries (CCRF) by FAO (FAO 1995) is voluntary, but impose moral obligation for governments to take steps to promote responsible and long-term sustainable fisheries. Article 7.4 states the need to consider scientific information to evaluate the state of fishery resources, need to disseminate results of research to interested parties and the need of timely, complete and reliable statistics on catch and fishing effort in accordance with applicable international standards and practices in sufficient detail to allow sound statistical analysis. FAO (2009) provided guidelines on information and knowledge sharing and its potential role in supporting implementation of the CCRF. These guidelines are inclusive of relevant principles, standards, practical suggestions, etc., for the enhancement of the role of the Code. Various issues involved in the flow of information between different stakeholder groups such as lack of information policy frameworks, ICT infrastructure, etc., are also covered. Webster and Collins (2005) identified the constraints in the effective implementation of the FAO Responsible Fisheries Code as lack of integration of publications generated in developing countries into the mainstream of fisheries and aquaculture information. Strategies for improving the capture, dissemination, sharing and preservation of fisheries information are also proposed.

General Literature: Fisheries

Ramakrishnan (2010) highlighted the concept of sustainable fisheries development and established the reasons for the failure of markets and governments due to the absence of proper information. According to him failed public policies built on un-sound information and knowledge; defunct social institutions without proper communication networks, etc were the serious constraints developing countries faced for natural resource management. The study also pointed out the need for information capacity building; co-management and use of traditional knowledge for the improvement and performance of the industry. Cochrane and Garcia (2009) in the collection of research papers edited by them emphasize the need for timely information for effective fisheries management. Information requirement for fisheries managers and decision-makers are discussed in detail in the collection under four domains namely (1) Biological (2) Ecological (3) Economic and (4) Social domains.

Malhotra and Sinha (2007) outline the growth, strength and weakness of Indian fisheries sector based on analysis of the primary and secondary data on fisheries and aquaculture collected from authoritative sources. The study examined the growth of fisheries sector against the backdrop of World Trade Organization (WTO) regime, globalization of world economies, liberalization of Indian economy and presented a comprehensive techno-socio-economic-political and legal review of Indian fisheries in the global context. Lack of reliable data of resources and production; serious gap between the availability of technologies and their dissemination; communication gap between the fishery scientists and the industry; need for development of extension materials, etc., have been stressed in the work.

Agarwal (2006) traced out history of fisheries in India from Vedic time to the present with stress to medieval and British Colonial period. Importance of fisheries and aquaculture, contributions of the sector to the national economy and other aspects of fisheries development in India, are discussed with support of statistics. Aruna and Pradhan (2006), in the paper titled 'Information and Communication Technology in Fisheries' in the 'Handbook of Fisheries and Aquaculture' discussed the application of information and computer technology in fisheries sector. It explained roles played by ICT for overall development of the sector.

Pillai and Katiha (2004) examined the aspects of evolution of fisheries research and development; aquatic resources and their production; fishing practices; post-harvest technologies; impact assessment and prioritization of technologies, etc. Dr S Ayyappan's (Director General, ICAR) foreword is notable with statements on inadequate documentation of fishery information, the highly scattered nature of management, options and possibilities relevant to each ecosystem/resource and the major handicaps to examine process of fisheries planning and development in the sector.

Ramachandran (2004) examined the management practices followed by the fisher folk and the concept of responsible fisheries endorsed to ensure sustainability of the resource in a system perspective. The extension system in the case of marine fisheries sector, confronted with a number of epistemological and methodological problems, needed to infuse new perspectives on re-inventing an extension system that can take a proactive role in creating ethos of responsible fisheries among stakeholders. The study suggests the need to transplant new theoretical developments in extension science like constructivism and social learning to the fisheries extension scenario with an extension paradigm. Study by Kochtanek and Matthews (2002) dealt with the role of standards in designing Library Information Systems, and stressed the need for professional involvement in developing standards that affect the dissemination of content to end users in increasingly complex technological environments. The study emphasized the need to be cognizant with the standards developed, the processes involved and the services delivered using new information technologies by the libraries.

Indian Institute of Management (1985) studied the parameters such as infrastructure facilities; market structure; distribution system; costs and margins; financial aspects; price-spread from consumer to fishermen; and infrastructure comprising of production and marketing in inland fisheries sector. As production and marketing are very closely interlinked, the study attempted to project fish supplies. The methodology developed for projecting supplies would be of interest to policy makers and others. The study also examined the state of the data and offered suggestions to strengthen this base. With regard to marine fish marketing in India, Indian Institute of Management (1984) published a detailed study report running into six volumes. It presented the situation in production and marketing of fish in eight maritime states of India. It gives projections of supply and demand for fish, infrastructure outlook and marketing channels. The study suggests for designing the Management Information System for improving interaction between the existing data collection agencies and its users.

Government of India (1976) in the Report of the National Commission on Agriculture-Part VIII: Fisheries described the fishing industry of India and discussed the trends and problems in the field of production, supply, demand, marketing, etc. It also gave a number of recommendations to promote the growth of the industry. Government of Kerala (1969) presented a brief account of the fisheries development in the State and a master plan for the future development of the sector which can be a reference document for fisheries information system designers and managers for developing relevant and need based systems and services in the sector.

General Literature: Library and Information Science

Mangala (2003) opined that in the present information age, developing and strengthening a country's information systems and infrastructures should receive high priority in the programmes of national development. A well-organized information system supported by an equally efficient information infrastructure would promote the information transfer more effectively and efficiently. A proper planning in each country would thus, greatly help in establishing National Information Infrastructure (NII). Satija (2003) asserted that despite the new technologies being increasingly adopted by libraries throughout the world, their fundamental mission to acquire and build a knowledge base, preserve documents of value, and provide value added information services in anticipation and on demand remains unchanged. He observed that digital technology could dramatically affect the nature of the information services.

Shakshuki, Ghenniwa and Kamel (2003) advocated for a new design paradigm for information systems with the fast growth of the information space in the Internet and large-scale Intranet computing environments. In such environments, the heterogeneity and the distributed nature of the information make it difficult for a user to locate and retrieve the desired information. Moreover, these computing environments being open, the information resources may join or disjoin at anytime and therefore, the study proposes a multi-agent multi-tier architecture. Agents being goal driven, they cooperatively assist different users to locate and retrieve information from distributed resources. Multi-architecture comprising three tiers, at the front end, the User Agents interact with the users to fulfill their needs. At the back end, Resource Agents access and capture the content of the information resources. At the middle tier, Broker Agents facilitate cooperation among the agents. A prototype of this system demonstrates that the agents can transparently cooperate to locate and retrieve information from dynamic and distributed information resources.

Metkewar and Acharya (2006) identified the need for Agricultural Information System by studying the information needs in agriculture in Marathwada region of Maharashtra. They recommend a modular approach constituting a sub-information system in different sub-systems of agriculture. The period of the study seems to be from 1970 to 2001. Ravisankar, Rajukumar and Shenbagakumar (2004) considered Open Access to agricultural resources, help desks, information centres, etc., as the highest priority to provide first hand information to farmers. Moni (2004) focused on the emerging areas in ICT and its role in sustainable agricultural development in India especially 'informatics led agriculture development' that can take India forward towards precision agriculture and enhancement of quality of life of the farming communities.

Sreenivasulu and Nandwana (2001) reviewed the networking of the Agricultural Information Systems and Services in India by covering a range of issues related to ARIS (Agricultural Research Information System) of ICAR; Agricultural Research Information System Network (ARISNET) and its modules; the strength and development of agricultural libraries in India including the institutional system of ICAR, State Agricultural Universities and ICAR institute libraries. Devarajan (2000) discussed the importance of agricultural information systems, and qualitative library and information services for agricultural development.

Raman Nair (2000) raised various concerns on information management, implementation and functioning of the ARIS under National Agriculture Technology Project (NATP) by ICAR. The study advocates that the personnel having specialization in Information Science should manage ICT units where information services are their mandate in agricultural sector. His study proved correct after a decade. ARIS was a non-starter. Though millions of rupees spent, ARIS could not put a single important agricultural research document in digital format in the web. Nevertheless, Deshmukh (1990) opined that the agricultural university libraries in collaboration with ICAR institutes should form a network of library and information system under the guidance of ICAR as technology transfer in agricultural sector needed a sound information base. However, ICAR could prove that effective services are beyond their imagination, the policy makers are beyond evolving right policies and the agency unable to apply relevant technologies. Nevertheless, ICAR made studies for improvement of libraries during initial years of development in independent India. Report of the Regional Agricultural Study and Survey Team sponsored by ICAR (1975) opined that the conditions of the libraries were not satisfactory and needed better information dissemination for quality education, research and extension. Dorothy Parker as Chairman, Indo-American Agricultural Library Survey and Study Team (1967) made recommendations for the improvement of the libraries of ICAR institutes and agricultural universities of that time. Ralph and Krishna

Rao (1956) Report could be considered as the first study of library and information services in agricultural sector, evaluating the library situation in agricultural education institutions and suggesting for improvement.

The survey of research on fisheries information sector of India revealed that only a very few deal specifically with fisheries information. Even those studies give superficial analysis and are devoid of any suggestion on specific framework, systems and services for flow of fisheries information to the stakeholders of the sector. There is hardly any study where perceptions of fishers, fish farmers and their community, entrepreneurs, hobbyists, marketers, financiers, traders, grass root level workers, NGO workers, extension workers, etc., are addressed. The major characteristic of the earlier studies is that they aimed at the improvement of information provisions to privileged few rather than the demand-driven, need-driven and time-driven information in the sector. Nevertheless, the reviewed studies have helped in formulating conceptual framework for the present study to some extent.

Though literature on Geographical Information Systems and Remote Sensing Systems in fisheries and aquaculture exist, services based on these technologies such as Preferred Fishing Zones (PFZ), Early Warning System, etc. are not readily disseminated on other information networks for use by fishers and farmers. Thereby, the primary stakeholders are often deprived and the informed people are benefitted in reaping public information services. There are also instances that farmers, extension workers and researchers are connected to networked community tele-services such as Information Villages Project of MS Swaminathan Research Foundation. Therefore an intensive study was necessitated by involving various representative libraries, information divisions, fisheries institutions, universities, government organizations, NGOs and private organizations at different levels, catering to a wide variety of user categories like scientists, extension workers, students, administrators, planners, fishers, fish farmers, etc. because a broad study only could address the problems in a holistic manner and suggest comprehensive, integrated and viable steps by applying state-of-the art concepts on ICT, resource sharing, networking and Information Management to ensure equal right and opportunity for fisheries information to all the stakeholders of the sector.

❑❑❑

Chapter-3

Conceptual Frame, Methods and Tools of the Study

What constitute Fisheries Information

According to FAO, fisheries information is characterized by four major features. (1) Fisheries information is broad and multidisciplinary (2) It has depth in terms of time and perspective (3) It involves various scales from very local to global and (4) It comes from a complex mix of sources (FAO 2009). Four types of information domains as per FAO (FAO 2005) are (1) Fishery and Operations (2) Biology and Environment (3) Economic and Financial and (4) Socio-cultural. For the present study, fisheries information denotes the aquatic and fishery information, too.

Conceptual Terms

The term 'Fishery' (plural fisheries) as defined by Webster's Dictionary in different contexts are (1) the business of catching, packing, or selling fish or other products of lakes, rivers, or the sea (2) a place where fish, etc are caught; fishing ground (3) the legal right to catch fish in certain waters or at certain times and (4) a place where fish are bred (Webster 1976). The term 'fisheries' is also used synonymously with 'fishing industry'. Royce defined fishery as a system composed of interacting components such as the aquatic biota, the aquatic habitat, and the human users of these renewable natural resources (Royce 1984). 'Sector' denotes the common term to group a broad array of economic activities that are in the same line of business (Olena 2006). The term 'sector' refers to distinct and large subdivision defined on the basis of some common factors.

Defining 'Information' is an elusive matter. Web defined 'Information' as the data (1) verified to be accurate and timely,

(2) specific and organized for a purpose, (3) presented within a *context* that gives it meaning and relevance, and (4) that can lead to an increase in understanding and decrease in uncertainty. (Business Dictionary 2010) The UNISIST-II (Main Working Document) gives a restricted meaning in the context of science, technology and societal development, as 'Information' is 'the symbolic elements used for communicating scientific and technical knowledge, irrespective of their nature (numerical, textual, etc) material carriers, form of presentation, etc. It refers to both substance and contents of documents and to physical existence; the term is also used to designate both the message (substance and form) and its communication (act)' (UNESCO 1979). According to Shannon and Weaver, information is 'the reduction of uncertainty'. (Crag 1999) As per Ratzan (2009), information is 'that which informs' and as per Ruben (1988), information is 'a coherent collection of data organized in a particular way that has meaning'. Information is 'the meaning that a human being assigns to data by means of the conventions applied to that data' (Stallings 1988).

'Information services' are helpful activities provided to user community to assist them in meeting their information needs and requirements. In simple terms, information service is a service which provides information in some way. Harrod's Librarians' Glossary and Reference Book defines information service as 'a service provided by a special library which draws attention to information possessed in the library or information department in anticipation of demand' (Prytherch 2005). Information service is an activity to find out what is already known on a particular subject or topic and make it available to the reader. Information service necessitates knowledge of the different varieties of information sources, their scope, characteristics and uses.

'Information resources' are the information assets of an agency or organization. University of Utah in its library regulations describe that 'information resources include any information in electronic, audio-visual or physical form, or any hardware or software that makes possible the storage and use of information'. This definition includes but is not limited to electronic mail, phone mail, local databases, externally accessed databases, CD-ROM, motion picture film, recorded magnetic media, photographs, digitized information, or microfilm. It also includes any wire, radio, electromagnetic, photo optical, photo electronic or other facility used in transmitting electronic communications, and any computer facilities or related electronic equipment that electronically stores such communications' (University of Utah 2013). The definition counts information resource as the assets of the library. Information resource itself is more like a piece of abstract information rather than a concrete document. The term is often used to refer to both abstract and concrete entity.

Measurements

Evaluating present status of fisheries information resources, services and system as a whole in different dimensions, quantitatively and qualitatively was one of the objectives of the study. According to Consultative Group on International Agricultural Research (CGIAR 1989), the emerging role of information resource management includes the planning, co-ordination and evaluation of all kinds of information resources within the sector. According to Horton (1974), "the main components of this process are the integration and harmonization of information resources, services and systems. The most important step in design of such systems is the preparation of an inventory of the three major resource categories namely information sources, services and systems". According to Bawden (1990) the goals of librarianship are collection, preservation, organization and access, and therefore the measurement/ quantification exercises for the study were mainly centered on the information capacities of the fisheries sector and on the goals of librarianship.

The resources and services chosen for this study are the information resources and services of all kinds pertaining to fisheries that are channelized through institutions in the fisheries sector. The study used a descriptive research design that involves instruments meant for collecting data for both quantitative and qualitative analysis of the resources and services. As part of the quantitative component, surveys and structured interviews were carried out, i.e., questionnaire by direct serving or e-mail as well as postal and face-to-face or telephone interviews. The qualitative analysis was done through in-depth interviews, focus group discussions, observation and field visits. In the light of the practical difficulties in measuring the process, effects and characteristics of fisheries information sources, services and systems in the sector by any single index, a series of causative and resulting indicators were formulated by consulting many sources on the subject. These indicators were used in the Questionnaires for evaluation processes.

Stakeholders

Four key stakeholders or partners in the sector are (1) Resource users (fishers); (2) Government (National, regional, local); (3) Other stakeholders (community members, boat owners, fish traders, boat builders, business people, fish farmers) and (4) Change agents (Academic and research institutions, development agencies, NGOs etc) (Pomeroy and Rivera-Guieb 2005). The LIS Professionals who serve all the above four stakeholder categories constitute the fifth estate in the fisheries information sector.

Characteristics of the Samples and Responses

The 'main stream institutions' constitute 15 National Fisheries Institutions, one Deemed University, one State Fisheries University and 18 Fisheries Colleges. They are classed as major institutions in fisheries sector because of the resources, infrastructure, functions, establishment and financial allotments they hold. There are also 22 National Institutions, 31 KVKs and 16 NGOs, Associations and Societies related to fisheries in India including those located in the Kerala State. They together cover all the subject areas related to fisheries sector. Detailed analysis was done for 15 National Fisheries Institutions, one State Fisheries University, 13 Fisheries Colleges and 11 National Institutions in the allied fields. Six National Fisheries Institutions are functioning in Kerala. There are nine State Fisheries Institutions and six out-stream State institutions functioning in Kerala. Minor institutions without planned information support systems come to six, excluding *Matsya Bhavans* and small cooperatives. Survey covered eight fisheries institutions including Universities/ Colleges of the State and five minor institutions including NGOs and Societies.

Indian fisheries research, education, extension and development system consists of approximately 800 scientists, 370 teachers, 195 researchers and 448 Post Graduate students in fisheries institutions including the sample State of Kerala. There are 20 LIS professionals working in National Fisheries Institutions and approximately another 25 working in Fisheries Universities and Colleges all over India. In the State of Kerala, three top level officers, 36 middle level officers and approximately 252 low level officers are employed in Department of Fisheries and allied agencies of Government of Kerala including *Matsya Bhavans*. Number of people working as extentionists and voluntary social workers in fisheries sector of Kerala are not known. As per statistics of the year 2008-09, there are 181015 active marine fishers and 54738 active inland fishers including women. They constitute 21% of fishermen population in Kerala. There are 113 Inland Fisheries Villages and 222 Marine Villages in Kerala (Government of Kerala 2009). Statistics with regard to people engaged in fish farming, trading and other allied operations and industries in fisheries sector in Kerala are not available.

Survey and interview were conducted among 538 users (84 Scientists, 55 Teachers, 46 Researchers, 89 Post Graduate Students, 44 Officers, 120 Fishers, 100 Fish Farmers, 17 Managers/Top Level officers, 14 LIS professionals, five Traders, five Entrepreneurs, five NGO/Extension Workers and three people's representatives) on all India basis to collect data considering the theme central to the nation and concurrent to the states of regional variations. There are hundreds of industrial firms in private sector in the State of Kerala. Institutions under government control were considered because of the 'public good' nature of fisheries information. NGOs and Associations are also included in the study considering their 'public welfare' activities.

Mixed methods of Survey using different types of questionnaire, interview, and field visits were used for eliciting data from respondents. The sample institutions were divided into four categories for the convenience of the study (1) National fisheries institutions, (2) State fisheries institutions, (3) Out stream national institutions and (4) Out stream State institutions based on their functions, resources, infrastructures and services. Out stream institutions constitute those functioning in the allied areas of fisheries sector such as rural development, management sciences, food sciences, nutrition, engineering, oceanography, earth sciences, aquatic sciences, remote sensing, ocean technology, etc,. All the National Fisheries Institutions, fisheries colleges situated in eastern, northern, western and southern parts of India, Universities, Departments, Colleges, institutions, NGOs and societies situated in Kerala constituted the sample institutions.

Respondent Group

The major stakeholders of fisheries sector are the scientists, teachers, researchers, students, planners, administrators, officers, peoples' representatives, NGO activists, extension workers, fishers, fish farmers, fish traders who need information and use information in their vocations and profit making. The different types of respondent groups are (1) Fisheries resource users i.e., Fishers, fishing community (2) Other stakeholders i.e., Fish farmers, boat owners, fish traders (3) Government i.e., Officials/planners/managers/people's representatives at national, regional, local levels of administration (4) Change agents i.e., Scientists, teachers, students (PhD and PG), researchers, officers, activists in education, research and development institutions, NGOs and (5) Library and Information Professionals in the national fisheries institutions/universities/colleges.

Sample Region

The study was carried out in the major national fisheries institutions, colleges and universities. Investigations of primary stakeholders, fishing villages and Department offices were conducted in the State of Kerala. With regard to Sample Size and Coverage, different types of users of fisheries information were included in the present study. Table 2 provides details of the research techniques adopted for data collection.

Sampling Design

Different sampling procedures were adopted for selecting the respondents. For Fisheries Resource Users i.e., Fishermen, the list of inland and marine fishing villages was prepared after consulting the data sources of Department of Fisheries, Kerala State. Two fishing villages from each category of inland and marine were selected from South, Central and North zones of Kerala State constituting three inland fishing villages viz., Vellayani, Thalayazham and Kumbalam and three marine fishing villages viz., Ambalapuzha, Chellanam and Vadanappally, respectively. For Selection of Respondents, in each selected village, households with fishers were identified and 20 respondents were selected using simple random technique. Thus, a total numbers of 120 samples were selected through systematic random sampling. For selection of respondents, the same procedure was adopted in both sets of villages.

Selection of Villages and Respondents

Fisheries development agencies namely Freshwater Fish Farmer's Development Agency (FFDA) and Aquaculture Development Agency in Kerala (ADAK), one each belonging to South, Central and North zones of Kerala viz., Alappuzha, Ernakulam and Thrissur were approached for the list of Registered Fish Farmers with address and contact details and 40 farmers were selected at random. List of registered Shrimp Farmers of Coastal Aquaculture Authority published in their Web site http://caa.org.in was consulted and 40 farmers belonging to different coastal districts were selected at random. Twenty numbers of farmers with e-mail address were selected at random from the Archive of Frequently Asked Questions in *Kissan Kerala* web site at www.kissankerala.net. Questionnaire in local language was sent by post and its English version by e-mail to farmers. Responses were collected directly by visiting Thalayazham and Kumarakom fishing villages for getting target number of responses to make up the deficiency caused by non-response by post and e-mail. For selection of Traders, Entrepreneurs and Allied Operators, marine fish landing centre at Vypeen and inland fish landing centre at Vaikom, major fish market at Fort Kochi and Champakkara, Small and Medium Enterprises (SMEs) on ornamental fisheries in Kumbalam and processing centres at Chandiroor were visited.

Table 2. Research Techniques Adopted for the Study

Method	Respondent	Instrument	Mode	Sample Selection
Survey	Librarians of National fisheries institutions	Questionnaire 1 on system resources and services	Post, e-mail, institution visit	Stratified. All responses from all the National fisheries inst.
Survey	Librarians of State fisheries Inst./Colleges universities/ NGOs	Questionnaire 1 on system resources and services	Post, e-mail, institution visit	Stratified. All responses from selected fisheries inst./universities/ colleges/NGOs
Survey	Information users: scientists, teachers, researchers, extensionists	Questionnaire 2 on system resources and services	Post, e-mail, institution visit	Stratified. All responses from all the National fisheries inst.
Survey	-do-	Questionnaire 2 on system resources and services	Post, e-mail, institution visit	Stratified. All responses from selected fisheries inst/ universities/ colleges/NGOs
Survey	Institution managers,	Questionnaire 3 on system	Post, e-mail, institution	Quota. All responses from all

	directors, senior scientists	requirements, plans, policies	visit	the National fisheries inst.
Survey	Institution officers, administrators	Questionnaire 3 on system requirements, plans, policies	Post, e-mail, institution visit	Quota. All responses from selected fisheries inst/ universities/ colleges/NGOs
Survey	Fish farmers, traders, entrepreneurs	Questionnaire 4 on information needs, use, access(in local language)	Local village/ home visit, Post, e-mail	Random. All respondents to Questionnaire 4
Survey	Fishers	Questionnaire 5 on information needs, use, access(in local language)	Local village/ home visit	Random. All respondents to Questionnaire 5
Interview	Scientists/ Officers in charge of inst/div/dept	Schedule on information capacity and views	Institution Visit	Judgment. Selection based on response to Questionnaire 2
FieldVisit	Libraries, Information Centres	Checklist on information resources, services and systems	Institution Visit	Observation. All the institutions visited

Selection of Fisheries Data Users in Planning, Administration, etc.

Organizational set up of the Department of Fisheries, Government of Kerala was verified and offices with diversified functions under the Department were identified as samples. The Selection of the Offices such as Matsya Bhavans at Muhamma, Mannar, Kumarakom, Vaikom and Udayamperoor; ADAK, Ernakulam; FFDA, Alappuzha, Ernakulam and Thrissur; Matsyafed, Trivandrum; Matsyafed, Thoppumpady; Joint Director of Fisheries (Central Zone) Ernakulam; Deputy Director of Fisheries (Ernakulam District), Ernakulam; Society for Assistance to Fisher Women (SAF) Kadungalloor; Fisheries Resource Management Society Kerala (FIRMA), Ernakulam; Fish Hatchery, Pannivelichira; Directorate of Fisheries, Trivandrum; Matsya

Grama Project, Trivandrum; Kerala State Coastal Area Development Corporation (KSCADC), Trivandrum and Kerala Fishermen's Welfare Fund Board (KFWFB), Thrissur were selected on systematic random sampling. For Selection of Respondents, twenty three officers at different levels of fisheries administration in the State of Kerala including 15 numbers of officers working at grass root level such as *Matsya Bhavans*, seven numbers of middle level officers functioning in Department and *Matsyafed* offices, and one top level officer at Directorate of Fisheries, Kerala State were selected as samples.

Selection of Fisheries Information Users in Education, Research, etc.

Under this category, Selection of Institutes comprised all the National fisheries institutions under ICAR and Ministry of Agriculture, Faculty/Departments of Fisheries/Aquatic sciences under Universities and Colleges of Fisheries located in different parts of India. All the institutions related to fisheries and aquatic sciences in Kerala State were selected for the survey and the study. Out-stream institutions at national and state level and NGOs of national and regional standing were selected at random as samples.

Respondents in these institutions constituted scientists, teachers, researchers, students and officers in the institutions. The percentage of responses was fixed at minimum 10 percentage of total strength of respondent categories selected for the survey. Care was taken to include the respondents from different streams such as research, education and extension; different departments in the institutions and different categories of users equally.

Selection of Libraries and Information Centres

Libraries and Information Centres of national fisheries institutes under ICAR, National Fisheries Institutions under Ministry of Agriculture, University Faculty/Departments of Fisheries/Aquatic Sciences, College of Fisheries located in different parts of India were selected to represent this category on national basis. Libraries in the institutes relating to fisheries and aquatic sciences located in Kerala state were selected to represent the State. Libraries in out-stream institutions on national as well as regional were also included. Respondents under this category constituted the Library and Information professionals working in fisheries libraries.

Period of Survey and Instruments of the study

The survey was carried out during the period from September 2011 to December 2012. The instruments used for data collection are:

- Structured questionnaire for LIS Professionals in the libraries of fisheries institutions.
- Structured questionnaire for scientists, teachers, officers, researchers and students.
- Structured questionnaire/interview schedule for Directors, Managers, Top officers of fisheries institutions.
- Structured questionnaire for fishers in the regional language (Malayalam).
- Structured questionnaire for farmers, traders and allied operators in the regional language (Malayalam).
- Observation.
- Field visits.

To ensure quality the following were adopted:

- Field visits by the researcher.
- Scrutiny of completed questionnaires and interviews.
- Proper and adequate preparations for interviews.
- Re-contacting the respondents after analyzing the responses.
- Re-checking and comparing data with information available in Annual Reports, brochures, etc.

The ethical issues were taken care of by:

- Conducting the research within stipulated standards.
- Informing the respondents on the purpose of the study.
- Taking informal consents prior to their participation in the study.
- Making systematic and data based enquiries during the survey and
- Ensuring honesty and integrity during the entire survey process.

Data Processing and Analysis

A pre-test was carried out with a proto type questionnaire and by interacting with the farmers, fishers, students and teachers. Inputs from them could help in formulating hypothesis for the study. A database for the respondents was created by collecting author affiliation addresses from journals, vernacular weeklies, dailies, proceedings of the symposia, home pages of various institutions, list of participants in various training programmes, etc., for communication and interaction. All the completed questionnaires were scrutinized at the field level before entering the data. Data entry was done using MS-Excel 2010 and the frequency of all variables was checked and the data was cleaned. The primary data was analyzed using Statistical Package for Social Sciences (SPSS Version 16.0) for determining Box plot and Chi-square test, to draw the inferences. The Chi-square test was used to determine whether there was a significant difference between the expected frequencies and the observed frequencies in the categories of ratings obtained from various groups of users. Kruskal-Wallis, one way of analysis of variance test was done to know significant differences in the ratings obtained from different respondent groups. Mann-Whiteney test was done to know whether there was any significant difference between two groups.

❑❑❑

Chapter-4

Fisheries Sector of India

'Fishery science' has two different meanings. First, it is a body of scientific knowledge pertaining to the fisheries and their environment. It is also called fisheries science or just fisheries. Second, it is a profession that expands and uses the body of scientific fishery knowledge to obtain optimum benefits for society from the living resources of the waters (Royce 1984). Thus, Fishery Science is a multi-disciplinary, multi-faceted and applied branch of knowledge. Scientific fisheries draw the basic principles not only from basic sciences such as botany, zoology, chemistry, physics and mathematics but also from disciplines of oceanography, geology, ecology, meteorology, aquatic biology, aquatic conservation, population dynamics, economics, management, sociology, statistics, engineering etc. Fisheries encompass a variety of sectoral spheres such as socio-techno-economic that are to be considered for systematic management involving management of natural resources, human resources and a variety of infrastructural installations and establishments (Sajeev Ghosh 2007).

The term 'fishery' comprises one or more stocks of fish, treated as a unit for the purpose of conservation and management. Fisheries include all activities related to the exploitation of fish that are categorized into two:

- Capture fisheries which are by far the most important and refer to the harvesting of natural fish stocks found in oceans, freshwater lakes, and rivers along with handling, marketing, processing and distribution of fish and fish products and
- Aquaculture which is performed in brackish coastal areas, irrigation reservoirs, canals, natural and man-made ponds, tanks, cages, pens and lagoons.

The Legacy

Fishing has been an important human activity for livelihood and sustenance since 90,000 years ago (palaeolithic period) (Yellen et al 1995). Fish and fisheries of India too, find a legacy of history, enduring tradition and mythological undertones, which dates back to 3000 BCE (Jhingran 1975). Fish occupies an important place in the Indian mythology, history and tradition. According to Hindu mythology, one of the incarnations of God was in the form of fish (*Matsyavathara*). Profuse references to fish are found in the great epics of the country, in the stone carvings and paintings. Various religious books in India dating back to Pre-Vedic, Vedic and Post-Vedic periods give voluminous information on different types of fishes, various aspects of their fishery biology, fishing gears, angling, fishery laws, etc (Agarwal 2006). Reference to fish, its trade and fisher community are also found in the Songs of the Sangam Age (1st to 4th Century CE) and in the diaries and records of travellers to India like Pliny and the anonymous author of the 'Periplus of the Erythrean Sea' early in the first century CE. Records also show that salt-fish trade flourished along the western coast of India during 18th century (Government of Kerala 1969). Traditionally, fishing has been the principal avocation for the livelihood of a segment of the population living in the coastal region, and on the banks of rivers, lakes and canals (Silas 1977).

Systematic attempt to study fish and fisheries of India can be traced back to the pre-independence era (Pillai and Katiha 2004). Post-independence era heralded organized development of Indian fisheries sector with a novel macro-economic support through succession of Five-Year Plans and establishment of chains of national and state level institutions catering to fisheries research and development (Panda 2009).

Importance of the Fisheries Sector

According to FAO figures, India currently occupies 3rd position in global fish production contributing about 4.18% of world fish production (Dehadrai 2006). India is the second largest in aquaculture production in the world (Government of India 2012A). The sector has high potentials for rural development, domestic nutritional security, employment generation, gender main-streaming as well as export earnings. Indian fisheries sector has been witnessing a steady growth, and the annual fish production has touched 7 million tons. The inland fish production has reached 4 million tons, i.e., almost doubled in the last decade. Fisheries and aquaculture contribute to nearly 1% of the Gross Domestic Product (GDP) and 5% of the agriculture and allied activities. The sector can provide livelihood for over ten million citizens at subsistence level of annual income (Planning Commission 2010).

India possesses more than 2 million sq. km. of Exclusive Economic Zone (EEZ) in the Indian Ocean alone, 14000 sq. km. of brackish water available for aquaculture and nearly 16000 sq. km. of fresh water lakes and ponds (Planning Commission 2001). India is also bestowed with a rich pool of fish germplasm. More than 10 percentage of global fish diversity is found in Indian waters. A total of 2163 species of finfishes have been recorded, out of which 157 (7.26%) inhabit upland cold waters, 454 (20.99%) in warm waters of the plains, 182 (8.14%) in brackish waters and 1370 (63.3%) in marine waters (Kapoor 2002). *FishBase* has listed 2384 finfish species from Indian subcontinent that includes 1704 marine, 762 freshwater, 202 endemic and 258 commercially exploited species (FishBase 2011). The vast resources of fisheries open up new frontiers of production and offer a challenging future for the programmes of research and development.

Disciplines under Fisheries Science

The subjects covered in fisheries science (Sinha 2005) are given in Table 3.

Table 3. Disciplines and Subjects under Fisheries Science

Discipline	Subjects
Fish Biology	Fish Taxonomy, Fish ecology, Fish disease, Fish genetics, Fish physiology, Fish reproduction, Fish endocrinology, Fish nutrition, Fish microbiology, Fish behavior, Fish biochemistry, Fish biotechnology.
Inland Fisheries	Fish Population dynamics, Aquatic ecology, Aquatic Chemistry, Culture based fisheries, Capture fisheries, Limnology and Reservoir fisheries, Estuarine/lagoon Fisheries, Cold water fisheries and aquaculture, Aquarium and sport fisheries management, Inland craft and gears, Freshwater aquaculture, Brackishwater aquaculture, Integrated fish farming, GIS.
Marine Fisheries	Marine biology, Marine fish biology and fish behavior, Fish population dynamics, Fisheries oceanography, Fishing technology, Sea farming, GIS.

Fisheries Economics& Statistics	Fisheries resource assessment and statistics, Fisheries natural asset accounting, Planning and evaluation, Resources economics, Fisheries cooperative, Finance management, Fisheries business management, Fisheries market forecasting and management. Socio-economics, Socio-anthropology.
Fisheries Extension	Inland fisheries extension, Aquaculture extension, Marine fisheries extension, Extension methodology, Fisheries communication and journalism.
Fisheries Engineering	Gear, crafts and engines, Aquaculture structures and implements, Electronics, Global positioning system, Fish passes, ladder and other fisheries facilities design and construction, Eco-restoration.
Fish Processing	Biochemistry and microbiology, Product development and value addition, Quality control and packaging, Management of freezing plants, cold storage and ice plants, Storage and transportation.
Fisheries Legislation	Environmental law, International fisheries legislation Common property aquatic legislation, Fisheries rules, acts and laws.
Fisheries Planning & Mgmnt	Research planning and management, Institution building and strengthening, Capacity building and Human Resources Development (HRD), Project preparation, monitoring and evaluation, Fisheries administration and governance

Principal Fisheries of India

The fisheries of India is broadly divided into (1) Marine Fisheries and (2) Inland Fisheries that can further divided into Culture Fishery, Stocking-cum-capture fisheries (Reservoirs) and Capture Fisheries. Inland fisheries resources consist of fresh water and brackish water. Capture fisheries consist of rivers and their tributaries and estuaries, lakes, etc., wherein fishes are harvested without having to sow the seeds. Culture fisheries comprise of ponds, tanks, swarms, marshes, etc wherein one has to sow the seeds, nurse it to proper size before harvesting. These segments have different settings, inputs and strategy. Comprehensive, timely and reliable information on the status of inland fisheries resources and production is extremely important for development planning at macro and micro levels.

The estuarine ecosystem, spread around the confluence of river and the sea, is acknowledged as the most productive aquatic environment harbouring an admixture of freshwater and marine biota. Important estuarine fisheries resources of India are Hooghly-Maltah estuary, Godavari estuary, Mahanadi estuary, Narmada estuary, Chilka lagoon, Pulicat lake and Kerala backwaters. There are 19370 reservoirs in the country covering an area of 3.15 million ha that comprises of small, medium and large reservoirs in the country (Sugunan 1995; Desai 2006; Gupta 2006). Floodplains and oxbow lakes of Ganga, Brahmaputra and Barak basins situated in the states of Uttar Pradesh, Bihar, Assam, West Bengal, Meghalaya, Manipur, Arunachal Pradesh and Tripura occupy important position in inland fisheries of India because of their magnitude and production potential and due to their importance as breeding and nursing ground for riverine fishes (Chitranshi 2006; Sinha 2006). Coldwater fisheries in upland lakes and man-made reservoirs have received little attention although they support a wide variety of aquatic fauna. In Indian uplands, 258 species of fish have been reported belonging to 76 genera of native and exotic ones that spread over Himalayan and peninsular plateau (Vaas 2006). The marine fishery resource of India is generally studied in five regions (1) Northwest (2) South-west (3) North-east (4) South-east and (5) Island fisheries. The marine fisheries in the territorial waters are managed by State governments and in the waters beyond up to the limit of EEZ by the Central government as per the provisions of Indian constitution (Schedule VII, Article 246, Entry 57 of List 1; Entry 21 of List II) (ICSF 2011).

Fisheries Development in India

Fishery cannot be considered in isolation from the life of the people and the political scenario of India (Randhawa 1986). Fishery history has a record of continuous developments and its successes and failures can guide the planning of fisheries. Indian fisheries and research activities remained dormant before independence. The contributions of early naturalists like Hamilton-Buchannan, Sykes, Jerdon, Gunther, Day, Alcock, Anderson and others who worked on the Indian aquatic fauna; systematics; distribution and bionomics of the fresh water and marine fishes are valuable. Hora, Misra, Trewaves, and others have also added to the knowledge of the ichthyofauna of the country (Agarwal 2006). Enactment of 'Indian Fisheries Act' in 1897 is considered as an important event in the history of Fisheries in India. The Act delegated to the States (erstwhile Provinces), the responsibility of development and conservation of fisheries in the inland and territorial waters of the respective States. It also empowered the States to formulate their own rules/laws for the safeguard of the fishery.

The Act provided certain conservational measures to prevent the destruction of the resources and therefore, the development, management and conservation of fisheries became principally a State subject (Silas 1977).

Notable 20th century studies on the fisheries of British India are by Sir FA Nicholson, Sir KG Gupta (Bengal Presidency), Dr James Hornell and Rao Bahadur V Govindan (Madras Presidency), Dr AT Sorky and Mr WH Lucas (Bombay Presidency). A report entitled 'Preliminary Guide to Indian Fish, Fisheries, Methods of Fishing and Curing' was published in 1941 by the Directorate of Marketing and Inspection giving an outline of the fishing industry in India. Based on the 'Memorandum on the post-war development of Indian fisheries' by the then Director of Zoological Survey of India, Dr Baini Prasad in 1943, two research institutions, the Central Marine Fisheries Research Station at Mandapam (later as Central Marine Fisheries Research Institute with headquarters at Cochin in 1971) and another one at Calcutta for inland sector (later renamed as Central Inland Fisheries Research Institute, Barrackpore) were established. Subsequently, Deep Sea Fishing Station (now Fishery Survey of India) was established at Bombay (Pillai and Katiha.2004).

Fisheries development and planning was undertaken through the Five-Year Plans formulated by the government. The initial Five-Year Plans, starting from the 1950s, focused more on the 'development' of the sector, and on increasing production, while it was only in the Ninth and Tenth Five-Year Plan period that the need for conservation and management was explicitly recognized (ICSF 2011).

Schemes and Agencies for Fisheries Development

Implementation of fisheries development schemes in India is in the purview of State governments. Therefore, the State governments are primarily responsible for the extension or transfer of technologies to the fishers and aquaculturists. Development schemes of the central sector are implemented by Central government through State Fisheries Department. Ministry of Agriculture is the apex body in the country for fisheries research and development. It has two departments namely (1) the Department of Agricultural Research and Education (DARE) and (2) the Department of Animal Husbandry, Dairying and Fisheries (DAHDF) to monitor and implement fisheries programmes. The former is responsible for agricultural research and education. ICAR is the nodal research organization and fisheries colleges under agricultural universities are the educational institutions.

Fisheries Research and Development

Concerted efforts for the development of the fisheries of the country were initiated on attaining independence in 1947. Establishment of the Central Fisheries Research Institutes for marine and inland fisheries, the Deep Sea Fishing Station, and subsequently, the Central Institute of Fisheries Technology were the steps taken for organized research and development of fisheries in India. Specialized research institutions were set up and organized research activities on multiple aspects of fisheries were gradually established under Five-Year Plans (Agarwal 2006). Freshwater Aquaculture Research and Training Centre established by CIFRI at Dhauli, Orissa became Central Institute of Freshwater Aquaculture (CIFA) in 1986. Simultaneously, Central Institute of Brackishwater Aquaculture (CIBA), Chennai and National Research Centre on Coldwater Fisheries (NRCCWF), now Directorate of Coldwater Fisheries Research (DCFR), Bhimtal were carved out from CIFRI to expand research activities on brackishwater aquaculture and coldwater fisheries, respectively. National Bureau of Fish Genetic Resources (NBFGR), Lucknow, established in 1983, is responsible for research on fish genetic resources of the country and conservation and preservation of fish germplasm.

Socio-Economic Development of Fishermen Communities

The fishing community occupies low status in the society. Several factors such as low social status, poor economic conditions, illiteracy, heavy leaning on middlemen, traditional fishing equipments and methods of fishing, low production rate and income influence the socio-economic conditions of fishermen (Silas 1977). Now, it is an accepted fact that the socio-economic advancement of the fishermen is essential for the proper development of the fishing industry. Flow of information and knowledge in a society is the pre-requisite for the sustainable socio-economic development. Fishing communities are no exception.

Non-Governmental Organizations (NGOs) In Fisheries

NGOs work at the grass-roots and motivate the people for their rights and privileges in the sector. Many NGOs fill in the gap where government institutions and departments fail. Nevertheless, government departments have not succeeded in creating an impact or to improve the quality of services they provide. This made the government to look towards NGOs to deliver services and make the people dependent on the NGOs (Bhose 2003). NGOs mainly work towards capacity building of the community by providing information, creating awareness and strengthening the capability of the people.

Women's Participation in Fisheries

In India, women population contributes substantially in the pre and post-harvest fisheries operations though they are not involved in active marine fishing. About 25% of the labour force in pre-harvest activities, 60% in export marketing and 40% in internal marketing are women. They are active in both artisanal fisheries and the commercial fishery sector and contribute substantially to both national and household food security (Dehadrai 2005). World Bank sources put women in the fisheries workforce as 72% in total work force of 10,316,000 (World Bank, FAO and WorldFish 2010). Traditionally, large numbers of women are involved in fish marketing in all the maritime states of India. Opportunities for women in fisheries could be enlarged in the field of integrated aquaculture, marketing and export as well as in research and technologies development. These opportunities could be heightened only through exchange of information and sharing of knowledge.

Fishery Resource Development

The fisheries resources have certain special features which have implications for development and management. The fisheries resources are living and self-renewing. They are of common property in nature but the fish catch is uncertain. Fish are wet, highly perishable and consist of discrete units of various size and shapes. It can rarely be processed at source. It presents technical problems in handling. Fishing is a hazardous occupation that requires special skills and equipment. According to Subba Rao, development is a technical aspect and for growth of the fishing industry, there need to imply information about the opportunities. In the primary sector, such information relates to location, distribution, resources, weather conditions, markets and technological matters. In the secondary and tertiary sectors, information is required about the availability of supply, seasonal variations in such supply, the consumer preferences, level of demand

and technological matters (Subba Rao 1986). Therefore, availability of the know-how and the personnel capable of utilizing the information are the important means for development of the sector.

History of Fisheries Administration

The oldest establishment in India was the Department of Fisheries formed in 1905 under the British State of Madras. Fisheries was considered as a provincial subject in the same manner as agriculture when the Indian Constitution 1935 came into force. Although States like Madras and Bengal implemented several schemes for the development of fisheries, other states though rich in potential resources, hardly paid any attention to the development of fisheries. But, the great Bengal famine of 1943 compelled the Central government to develop the fisheries on an all India basis. The Government of India decided that some central agency was necessary to advise and coordinate development in the various sectors of fisheries. A section of Fisheries Development was created and attached to the Ministry of Agriculture. The Advisory Board of the Indian Council of Agriculture Research in its Memorandum of 1944, generally known as the Kharegat Memorandum laid down some of the essential directions to achieve fisheries development in the country. Report of the Fish sub-committee of the Policy Committee on Agriculture, Forests and Fisheries 1945 recommended to embark comprehensive programmes on (1) survey of fishing area, (2) initiation and coordination of research, (3) conservation, development and exploitation of fisheries, (4) improvement of the socio-economic conditions of the fishermen, (5) provision of more efficient and modern crafts and (6) organization of the fish trade on proper lines. Suggestions of Hornell and Swell in 1947 formed the basis for the establishment of the two Fisheries Research Stations of the Central government (Pillai and Katiha 2004).

Fisheries Management

Fisheries management is the process that has evolved to ensure that fisheries operate in a manner that not only provides the immediate benefits but also does not result in excessive or irreversible damage to the exploited fish stocks or the diversity, integrity and structure of the ecosystem, so that the stocks and ecosystem will continue to provide the full range of benefits in the future. The concept of fisheries management has assumed importance due to the diminishing fishery resources all over the world due to unsustainable practices observed in the fisheries sector. The FAO Code of Conduct for Responsible Fisheries has given further impetus to the fisheries management. Table 4 categorizes the data requirements for fisheries managers and decision-makers as per FAO Tech Guidelines 1997 (Cochrane and Garcia 2009).

Table 4. Data Requirements for Fisheries Management Functions

No	Objective	Data requirements
1	Biological	Stock structure; Total landings by major species or stock units per fleet per year; Total efforts by fleet per year; Length and / or age composition of landings, by fleet, for major species; Discards of species per fleet per year; Length and /or age composition of discards per species of particular interest per fleet per year; Areas fished by each fleet; Life history parameters; Abundance trends
2	Ecological	Total catches of by-catch species (including discarded species),or selected indicator species, per fleet per year; Length and/or age composition of catches of by-catch species or selected indicator species; Impact of fishing gear and activities on the physical habitat; Impact on critical habits brought about by non-fishery activities; Impacts of non-fishery activities on other components or Properties of the ecosystem
3	Economic	Average income per fishing unit per year for all fleets; Costs per fishing unit per year; Profitability of each fleet; Destination of landings from each fleet, and a measure of the dependence on the fishery of other sectors of the community
4	Social	Total number of fishers employed within each fleet; Total Number of people employed in fishing or shore-based activities per fleet, by gender and age group where appropriate; Dependence of fishers and shore-based workers for their livelihoods

Fisheries Governance

The term governance is synonymously used with management. Modern fishery governance is a systemic concept relating to the exercise of economic, political and administrative authority. Fishery governance establishes the over-riding principles and objectives of the sector. It develops the policy and regulatory frameworks. It connects government with civil society by harmonizing individual, sectoral and societal perspectives and maintaining social order and productive socio-ecological systems. Fishery governance has international, national and local dimensions. It includes legally binding rules, such as national policies and legislation or international treaties as well as customary social arrangements. It is multi-scale, covering long-term, strategic planning as well as short-term operational management and local fisheries as well as whole ecosystems. It has public, private, and hybrid components that interact in ensuring administration and regulation of the sector (FAO 2001).

The benefits and deficiencies of stakeholder participation in fisheries governance is now a lively debate (Tim 2005). The participatory mode of fisheries governance is based on effective communications that are able to bring together the viewpoints of many stakeholders so that management decisions can be generated (Wilson and Delaney 2005). Thus, the decision making hierarchy could make possible both a richer knowledge base and greater public support for management decisions with flow of information.

In India, governance of fisheries and marine habitats is spread across several agencies and Ministries at the Central level viz., Department of Animal Husbandry, Dairying and Fisheries; National Fisheries Development Board; Coast Guard (Ministry of Defense); Ministry of Environment and Forests (MoEF); Earth Commission (Ministry of Earth Sciences) and Planning Commission of India. Several conservation measures have also been initiated by the MoEF, especially towards safeguarding against trade in endangered species, protection of certain habitats such as coral reefs, mangroves and breeding grounds of turtles, by designating protected areas (ICSF 2011). Community-level institutions also play an important role in fisheries governance in Indian coast. '*Kadakodi*' system of Northern Kerala, '*Pedhaloo*' in South Odisha, traditional Panchayat system of the *Pattanavars* community of Tamil Nadu-Andhra Pradesh coast are some of the traditional governance systems (Ramachandran 2004). Bodiguel *et al* (2009) opine that good governance provides access to information and decision-making to legitimate stakeholders and interested parties in order to decrease vulnerability to cronyism and politically favouring some short-term interests over other, often long-term interests.

Traditional Knowledge in Fisheries Governance

Traditional Knowledge (TK) is not something new or innovative but the distillation of practices or knowledge in the society. TK is generally small-scale, qualitative and empirical knowledge and often anecdotal. Scientific fisheries information is generally large-scale, quantitative and rational, largely statistical, ostensibly objective, apparently universalistic, and highly systematic. Often, there is a stand-off between these two irreconcilably different forms of knowledge. Because of the failures of contemporary science-based fisheries management, there is an increasing acceptance of Traditional Fisheries Knowledge (TFK) as the dominant guide for fisheries managers (Johannes 2003).

It is important for communities to protect Traditional Knowledge. Individuals who are intimately associated with the resource have a wealth of knowledge that can enhance research and improve management (Stanley and Rice 2003). India has experienced various initiatives regarding the protection of TK under Intellectual Property Rights, including the Traditional Knowledge Digital Library (TKDL) which is a major step to curb bio-piracy. India has taken misappropriations of its traditional knowledge by developed countries through patenting system (Hirwade and Hirwade 2012). Though India has taken up traditional knowledge with respect to Turmeric, *Neem* and *Basmati* Rice, similar efforts in fisheries sector are not forthcoming.

Scientific Advice in Fisheries Governance

Science is defined as the 'systematized knowledge derived from observation, study, and experimentation carried on in order to determine the nature or principle of what is being studied (Webster 1976). Science provides a body of knowledge and a mechanism for answering questions posed by society. The questions likely to concern in the context of fisheries are the possible configurations of the exploited system and how to manage the system. The management of fisheries and resources is the responsibility of policy-makers and administrators, but it is generally agreed that sound management measures must be based on proper scientific advice. Sahrhage (1992) argues that the situation puts considerable responsibilities on to the scientists as well, not least in view of the great economic and political implications.

Sustainability in Fisheries Development

According to United Nations (1987) 'sustainable development' denotes the development that meets the needs of the present without compromising the ability of future generations to meet their own needs. Kelly (1992) elucidates that sustainable development uses a number of old concepts in new ways to address new problems and marries them with the relatively new biological science of ecology to provide developmental solutions. Jha (2004) says it is a synthesis of economic and ecological ideas that refers to creating a style of economic development which is sustainable within the context of the planet's eco-system and human society.

For sustainable development, information on bio-ecological component of the fishery system is necessary. Though considerable information is available, it may not be adequately interpreted, cross-linked, nor are the connections with policy development and fishery management planning appropriate. The lack of appropriately interpreted and cross-linked information is considered an impediment to convincing decision-makers. Currently, national and regional development organizations focus more on overall development issues than on individual sectoral programmes. The 'infoDev Programme' of the World Bank (2008) recognizes the importance of sharing information to plan and promote sustainable development.

The Code of Conduct for Responsible Fisheries (CCRF)

The CCRF was unanimously adopted by FAO Members on 31 October 1995 to which India is a member. Although a voluntary instrument, compliance with the Code is one of the most important processes to assess the performance and sustainability of the fisheries and aquaculture sector at global level. The ecosystem approach to fisheries (EAF) and ecosystem approach to aquaculture (EAA) are holistic strategies for managing capture fisheries and aquaculture that integrate their ecological, socio-economic and institutional dimensions and facilitate sustainable use of natural resources and integration with other users of coastal ecosystems (FAO 1995). Soto *et al* (2012) opine that to enhance the implementation of an ecosystem approach to fish production whether from wild catch or from farming, there is a need for capacity building at national and local levels and it is necessary to develop, access and improve practical tools that are in tune with local needs and capacities.

The CCRF recognizes that reliable and timely data are required for the competent authorities of national governments to effectively discharge their general responsibility in the promotion of sustainable aquaculture practices that are well integrated into rural, agricultural and coastal development (FAO 2005). Much of the Code refers to the development and wise use of knowledge. Every article of the code exhorts States, organizations and individuals to collect data, develop knowledge and apply appropriate measures for dissemination and sharing of information.

Fisheries Laws and Regulations

The Indian Parliament enacted the Territorial Sea, Continental Shelf, Exclusive Economic Zone (EEZ) and other Maritime Zones Acts in 1976. EEZ of 200 nautical miles is effective from January 15, 1997. For the judicious exploration, exploitation, conservation and management of marine living resources the Government has also enacted legislations viz:

- Marine Products Export Development Authority Act 1972.
- The Wild life Protection Act 1973 and various central legislations on environmental protection.
- Indian Coast Guard Act 1978 and
- The Maritime Zones of India (Regulation of Fishing by Foreign Fishing Vessels) Act 1981.

Under the enabling provisions of the Indian Fisheries Act, 1897, various States and Union Territories have introduced their fishery regulations. For regulation of fisheries in the territorial waters, all the coastal States and the Union Territory of Lakshadweep (except Gujarat and the remaining Union Territories) have enacted their Marine Fishing Regulation Act (MFRA) based on a model bill provided by the Union Government in 1979. The MFRA by the maritime provincial governments and the deep sea fishing schemes as provided under the Maritime Zone of India (Regulation of Foreign Fishing Vessels) Act, 1981 of the Government of India provide for prohibition of fishing by foreign vessels in the areas earmarked for the traditional and small motorized crafts. However, at present there is no law to regulate Indian owned deep sea fishing vessels. Besides effective and implementable legislation to regulate fishing by the Indian owned fishing vessels in the EEZ and compliance of international agreements (Straddling Stock Compliance Agreement), legal support is also necessary to regulate various production functions (e.g. fin and shell fish seed); domestic and international trade (e.g. standards for hygiene and product specifications); movement of live aquatic animals within the country and from across the borders (e.g. Quarantine) and conservation of resources and germplasm (e.g. revision of MFRAs) (ICSF 2013). A sound regulatory framework developed in consultation with the community stakeholders and integrated with information systems shall pave the way for compliance of laws and regulations in the country.

Indian marine fisheries coupled with open access regime and unplanned expansions of fishing efforts have been detrimental to the marine fisheries. Symptoms of unmanaged fisheries like recruitment and growth, overfishing, fishing down to food web and decline of charismatic species are also reported (Bhathal 2004). Enforcement enabled legislation support, mandatory installation of by-catch reduction devices as well as a viable and pragmatic fishing vessel monitoring and surveillance system can only reverse the downward trend for which an information system operable through extension, enforcement and outreach segments of fisheries sector is necessary.

Fisheries Economics, Industry and Marketing

Fisheries consists of complex societal constructions involving socio-economic issues, economic reforms, new trade regimes, rural finance, co-operatives, marketing, food quality and other special characteristics of fisheries resources. According to Anderson (2011), fisheries economics effectively combine the tools and perspectives of biology with those of economics to produce improved economic outcomes for consumers and people involved in harvesting, raising, processing and marketing fish. Fisheries economics also associate economic outcomes with the management characteristics. Fisheries also need a thorough back-up of scientific and management information. Economic benefit accrues to stakeholders when timely available information is put to productive use.

By and large, the fishing industry of the country is in the private sector. This includes the traditional fishing industry as practiced by the small-fishermen, small partnership or limited companies and large business houses (Silas 1977). The investment, operation and management vary in these fisheries establishments. The traditional sector of the fishing industry is in an unorganized state and the industry under the companies and larger houses are fairly well organized. Fisheries cooperative federations of the State governments, central fisheries corporations and state fisheries corporations promote marketing. These agencies do not have any direct links with production units/cooperatives. An efficient marketing information system for better management of the catch and distribution is also absent in the sector.

Aquaculture

Aquaculture is variously defined as 'fish farming' or 'husbandry of fish and shellfish'. FAO (2012) defined aquaculture as 'the farming of aquatic organisms, including fish, crustaceans, mollusks, and aquatic plants'. It implies farming as 'some form of intervention in the rearing process to enhance production, such as regular stocking, feeding, and protection from predators, etc. Farming also implies individual or corporate ownership of the stock being cultivated'. Aquaculture is recognized only recently in 2001 as an independent economic activity by the United Nations Statistical Commission. Accordingly, the collection of statistical data and other information on aquaculture separately from other fisheries data is a recent endeavor at the national, regional and global levels.

Fish farming is an effort to manage a biological process but capture fishery is beyond control. If fishing can be equated to hunting activity, aquaculture is agriculture, cultivating fish in a fixed location. Like the crop producer, the fish farmer has to be concerned with the growth and timing of the harvest. Fishing entails only harvesting, the rest taken care of by nature itself. Thus, knowledge of fish physiology and biology is vital to fish farmers whereas capture fishers function without knowledge of these aspects. However, technologies and knowledge of operation of gears are vital in aquaculture as well as in fishing. The fishers and the fish farmers are equally concerned once their product is harvested especially information relating to marketing and other allied operations. Therefore, aquaculture is not only a technical and biological innovation, but also a socio-economic enterprise that requires the same kind of social analyses as any other production system (Venugopal 2005) which is fairly information dependent. Alongside the 'Make in India' initiative launched by the government of India, there ought to be as well a 'Grow in India' initiative predicted on market reforms for the agricultural sector which empower producers and consumers rather than middlemen.

Ornamental Fish Industry

Ornamental fishery provides job and business opportunities for many in the culture and trade sector. Breeding and culture of ornamental fishes could generate great employment in rural India. Proper dissemination of information can entail ornamental fishery into a thriving industry. India has some of the finest ornamental fishes in the seas as well as inland waters. But, the trade should not be based on exploitation of naturally occurring stock but a well planned breeding system.

Trade Regimes

Malhotra and Sinha (2007) state the need for detailed knowledge about fishery sector as India has assumed importance with the establishment of World Trade Organisation, signing of World Trade Agreement and the globalization of world economies. The Chennai Declaration of the MSSRF-FAO Expert Consultation emphasize that the future of Indian agriculture depends on three factors viz., research, public policy and the farming community's cooperative action (MSSRF 2001). Therefore, the greater the synergy among these three factors, the better it would be for India. Research does not mean merely laboratory research; it includes research that would inform policy in all its aspects. Scientific organizations need to work with farmers and fishermen to move food security and nutrition higher up in the political agenda. Much of life sciences and agricultural research is coming under proprietary science and Subbaih and Umarani (2001) caution that unless India gears up publicly funded agricultural research, there is the imminent danger of long-term dependence on multinational corporations for knowledge, when agriculture is increasingly becoming knowledge intensive.

A large number of ancillary industries such as ship-building, marine engines, nylon manufacturing, net making, rope making, freezing, canning, fish meal, fish oil, cold storage, ice manufacturing, etc., comprise of fishing industry. Therefore, the revenue potentiality of fisheries is significant. Information on the various aspects of fisheries economics has seldom appeared in literature. Though much research work has been done in the biological and marine sciences, it is not properly coordinated with the economic theory. Organized information on the social and economic components of the fishery system is also seldom available.

Geographic Information System (GIS) in Fisheries

Fisheries management and planning has many spatial components and issues in fisheries like habitat loss and environmental degradation. GIS technology can be of great help to clarify the issues and to find solutions by treating many spatial components simultaneously (Geoffery and Thang 1996). GIS technology integrates common database operations such as query and statistical analysis with the unique visualization and geographic analysis (Clarke 1986). According to Raghu Prakash (2009) the major areas of application of GIS in fisheries include:

- Marine water conditions and habitats.
- Natural marine resources.
- Fisheries management – resource allocation and regulation.
- Fishing effort and catches.
- Marketing of fishery products.
- Mariculture and
- Coastal zone management.

Developments in GIS technology could enhance the capabilities of GIS as a tool for decision support for fisheries management and in explaining events, predicting outcomes and planning strategies for sustainable fisheries development.

Remote Sensing in Fisheries

Satellite remote sensing plays an important role for location of Preferred Fishing Zone (PFZ) and management of fishery resources by providing synoptic measurement of oceanic parameters such as sea surface temperature and colour (Somvanshi 2002). As the inland fisheries resources are vast, varied and scattered across the country, enumeration of these resources through conventional methods for developing reliable baseline data is rather impossible. Remote sensing techniques are quick, reliable and cost effective and can efficiently used in mapping and assessing the total water spread area of the country. Information on features such as fronts, eddies, gyres, currents and upwelling derived from satellites is useful in fisheries (Choudhury et al 2007). Dissemination of remotely sensed information to the fishers is vital for the utilization, ensuring profits and judicious exploitation of resources. Fishermen also require accurate weather forecasts, warning and advisory services for their living.

Constraints in Fisheries Development

Fisheries and its development is a major component of planning for a socialistic pattern of society. The planning and development of socio-economic conditions of fishermen vis-a-vis the resource management requires a considerable amount of information as to the demographic and socio-cultural characteristics of fishing communities, their occupational structure, income levels and other indicators of well being, the size of resource base, productivity, cost structure and profitability of existing technologies, the efficiency of marketing system, social and institutional constraints (Sankar Rao and Raju 1998). Flow of information is vital for aquaculture development also since aquaculture is interdisciplinary by nature. The two world conferences on aquaculture, viz., the Food and Agriculture Organisation Technical Conference on Aquaculture held in Kyoto, Japan in 1976 (FAO 1976) and World Conference on Aquaculture in Veniece, Italy in 1981, highlighted the importance of (1) technology development and improvement through research, (2) training of personnel and (3) information dissemination for rapid and orderly development of the sector (Bilio, Rosenthal and Sinderman 1981).

The major factors identified as potential constraints in fisheries development in India are (1) Data base on resource availability (2) Infrastructure facilities (3) Promotion and marketing support (4) Transport (5) Financing for vessels and marketing (6) Licensing/ leasing/Taxation procedures (7) Seeds (8) Feed (9) Extension and (10) Support services etc (NCAER 2010). At present, there is no focused policy on the fisheries sector. The Agricultural Policy announced by the government contains only a passing reference regarding the fisheries development in the country (Anjani Kumar et al 2003). Draft Marine Fishing Policy submitted to the government in 2002 is not promulgated as policy. However, the theme of comprehensive marine fishing policy is enshrined in the National Agriculture Policy promulgated by the Government (Malhotra and Sinha 2007). Considering the potential and prospects of fisheries and aquaculture development in the country, strategies for the implementation of the National Aquaculture Development Plans have been formulated (Agarwal 2006). The Plan underpinned the need to strengthen fisheries information sector in the country.

National Information Policies and Practices

The policy defines an area within which a decision is to be made and ensure that decisions will be consistent with, and contribute to an objective (Koontz and Weihrich 1990). Information policy is a set of interrelated principles, laws, guidelines, rules, regulations and procedures guiding the oversight and management of the information life cycle - the production, collection, distribution/dissemination, retrieval and retirement of information (Duran 1991).

According to UNISIST-II Main Working Document, 'A National Information Policy is a set of decisions taken by a government, through appropriate laws and regulations, to orient the harmonious development of information transfer activities, in order to satisfy the information needs of the country. A national policy needs provision of necessary means/instruments (financial, personnel, institutional) for concrete implementation' (UNESCO 1979).

In India, the need for harnessing information to support various activities relating to planning, policy-making, executive functions and other types of implementation processes; are recognized by the Government. A variety of institutions dealing with information are also established. In their development, these institutions have sprung up in a rather piecemeal way, without any plan of coordination and without a framework for leading to an integrated national system. Despite the thinking and executive actions of the Government at different stages, endorsing the fact that information is a vital resource worthy of care, harnessing and management, positive guidelines from the Government for a harmonious development of a versatile, integrated information system for the country, encompassing the information requirements of all sections of the society, are still lacking (Rajagopalan and Rajan 1986).

The objective of a National Information Policy is to achieve a progressive up-lift in the socio-economic development of the country through the provision of information and its effective use. Although a National Information Policy is required to bring into focus the imperativeness of this situation, it is yet to be formulated in India. The ultimate purpose of information is to put knowledge to work, and in turn, to improve the quality of life of the people. This fact is re-emphasized in the Report of the National Knowledge Commission, 2006 charged with considering possible policies that might sharpen India's comparative advantage in the knowledge-intensive service sectors. For utilization of information and knowledge in fisheries sector, sectoral information policy has to be construed. The policy formulated thus, should be followed by a sequence of activities viz., procedures, rules, programmes and budgets.

Fisheries Information Domains

Information domains as per FAO (2005) are:

- *Fishery and Operations*: all aspects of the primary capture of aquatic resources and their processing; who caught what amounts of fish, when and how; and what operational management information is required.
- *Biology and Environment*: all characteristics of the biology, dynamics and interactions of exploited living aquatic resources and their associated species within the biological and physical framework of the ecosystem.
- *Economic and Financial*: all aspects of the conduct of the fisheries sector, including human resource, financial and economic, and production and trade issues.
- *Socio-cultural*: all features that are needed to evaluate fisheries policy and management in relation to distribution of income and food, equity and demographics, and participant dependence and social status.

Fisheries Information Sources

Libraries are the storehouse of knowledge and they function as the pivotal agencies for providing information. Therefore, information capacities are measured through library and information resources, systems and services operating in the sector. 'Sources' does not merely imply document resource but an information product delivered either by individuals or organizations which furnish information and data to users (Satyanarayana 1993). Library might be considered as the location or person from where the user can obtain the information he requires.

International Fisheries Information Resources related to India

FAO is the only intergovernmental organization that maintains global fisheries statistics. The FAO, ever since its inception in 1945 continuously publishes a wealth of information across a very broad subject range. It has been instrumental in promoting fisheries development in the less developed countries of the world (Korakandy 1994). Silas (1977) aptly commented that various programmes and activities of FAO have benefitted the country in finding solutions to the urgent problems encountered and the overall development of fisheries of the region.

Publications that are of regular series category are FAO Fisheries and Aquaculture Technical Papers, FAO Yearbook of Fishery and Aquaculture Statistics (1947 onwards) and the Technical Guidelines for Responsible Fisheries. They are distributed worldwide. The State of World Fisheries and Aquaculture (SOFIA) the flagship publication of the Department, is published every two years. SOFIA is the premier advocacy document to provide policy-makers, civil society and the stakeholders a comprehensive, objective and global view of capture fisheries and aquaculture (FAO 2002). Other regular series such as FAO Fisheries and Aquaculture Circulars, Technical Papers are the quicker means of spreading fisheries information. Reports of FAO fisheries projects, papers presented at many FAO technical meetings etc, often referred to as 'grey literature' are also published. Global time series are maintained over 50 year time spans. FishStat Plus –the universal software for fishery statistical time series provides users with access to Fishery Statistics of various sorts. FishStatJ, a Java-based desktop application, is the new generation of the FishStat Plus software (FAO 2013). The challenge of distribution of bibliographic data for all FAO Fisheries publications and documents via the FAO on-line catalogue or via international databases such as ASFA, has effectively been met with information technology.

Besides FAO, there are number of fisheries information resources. Appendix 5 discusses International Institutions and web resources. Appendix 6 discusses Fisheries Information Services and Products for finding fisheries information. The World Database in Agriculture (World Database Series), Edited by Armstrong, C.J, published in 1996 by Bowker-Saur., London lists the World Databases in Aquatic and Fisheries Science from page 321to 347. It gives details of all the types of databases in various formats available then.

Fisheries Statistical Information

The inadequacies of database and anomalies in the available data had been a matter of concern in the planning and decision-making process in fisheries sector. Biradar (2000) states it as one of the reasons for the failure of the long-standing efforts of fishery management. The need for compilation of accurate, relevant and timely data in standard form facilitates monitoring, comparison and analysis of status and trends. Sound database on socio-cultural and economic aspects are also essential in order to avoid social conflicts among fishermen. Statistics based on well designed survey on market statistics and socio-economic are also required. Database on availability of inputs such as gears, crafts, feed, seed, fertilizer along with price, subsidy also need to be developed. There is also a need for online database on international market trend to the seafood exporters of our country. Up-to-date information on shrimp farming operations including water quality and other environmental parameters will provide the basis for control and monitoring of shrimp farming sector.

National fisheries data are periodically released by Government of India, Fisheries Division, Ministry of Agriculture and Cooperation in the form of Handbook of Fisheries Statistics providing information on fish production, export of marine products, fishing harbours, outlays and expenditure, prices, fishery resources, international comparison and schemes implemented for fisheries development etc. The handbook also contains data on infrastructural facilities, fishermen population, fish seed hatcheries, disposition of fish catch as fresh, dried, frozen, cured, canned, reduced etc.

The Central scheme on 'Strengthening of Database and Information Networking for the Fisheries Sector' is aimed to improve the database of inland and marine fisheries resources and catch of fish by adopting standardized methodology of data collection. It also aims to improve Information Technology System in the States/UTs as well as National fishery institutes so that data collection and their analysis can be one efficient and effective. Marine Fisheries Census 2010 is published by CMFRI (Government of India 2012). IndiaStat.Com is India's comprehensive statistics information portal that provides recent, exhaustive, authentic socio-economic statistical analysis and time-series data for all the major socio-economic parameters of the Indian States. It is a cluster of 51 sites including India-specific, sector specific and State specific sites rendering dedicated services to the research fraternity from academic, professional and corporate world with authentic and comprehensive compilation of secondary level socio-economic statistical data on more than 35 variables including fisheries statistics. MPEDA publishes statistics of marine products exports with details of major markets for marine products from India, country-wise, item-wise and port-wise.

Fisheries Research Information

The fisheries research in India is coordinated by the Fisheries Division of the ICAR. Mission of the Division is 'sustainable growth of Indian fisheries and aquaculture by interfacing research, education and extension resulting in a proper fit between the human needs and the habitat, with an important role in global fisheries'. The mandates of the Division are to formulate and supervise council's policies and works pertaining to fisheries research; to coordinate and stimulate operational research programmes and demonstration in different fisheries systems; and to serve as knowledge repository and clearing house in fisheries sector. Documenting entire information on fisheries and aquaculture in the country for providing inputs to policy and governance also forms the main objective of the Division (ICAR 2012). The ICAR has established eight different resources specific fisheries research institutes for developing technologies for exploitation and conservation of fisheries resources of freshwater, brackishwater, coldwater, coastal and marine ecosystems, and for harvest and post-harvest technologies, and an exclusive fishery institute for human resources development.

Fisheries Education Information

The ICAR has been playing a significant role in the field of agricultural education as the University Grants Commission (UGC) does in the general education. The aim of fisheries education and training in India is to develop skills and proficiency to increase the fish production through resource assessment, improved fishing techniques, handling, preservation, distribution and utilization by applying modern know-how, and by efficient management for achieving greater profitability and also for the social advancement of the fishing community. Fisheries education and training in India has four levels (Silas 1977; Biradar 2006):

- Base level: Operative technical personnel for the artisanal fisheries. Fishermen Training Centres, *Krishi Vigyan Kendras* and Trainees Centre of ICAR, Inland fisheries training centres under the State governments, etc. work at the Base level.
- Under-graduate level: Statutorily required personnel for manning ocean going fishing vessels, trained personnel for handling,

processing and marketing of fish, shore-based personnel for fabrication of fishing gear, maintenance of vessel, machinery etc. CIFNET was established to conduct regular training courses to create certificated officers for manning modern ocean going fishing vessels with skippers and engineers as per the provisions of the Indian Merchant Shipping Act, 1958.

- Graduate level: Development and managerial personnel to plan and to be in-charge of developmental programmes and
- Post-Graduate level: Scientific and technical personnel for stock assessment, exploration, introduction of new technology etc.

The Zoology Departments in Indian universities also impart fisheries education and research programmes. As on 22 Jun 2012, there are 568 UGC approved Central (4), State (285), Deemed (129) and private (113) universities in India (Wikipedia 2012). Over 400 Universities conduct education and research in biology, aquatic biology, pure and applied zoological sciences. The University of Agra (Uttar Pradesh), Annamalai (Tamil Nadu), Mumbai (Maharashtra), Veer Narmad South Gujarat University (Gujrat), Goa (Goa), Andhra (Visakhapatnam), Osmania (Andhra Pradesh), Bhavnagar (Bhavnagar), Burdwan (West Bengal), Culcutta (West Bengal), Kalyani (West Bengal), Viswa Bharti (West Bengal), Cochin University of Science and Technology (Kerala), Kerala (Kerala), Mahatma Gandhi University (Kerala), Calicut (Kerala), Madras (Tamil Nadu), Meerut (Uttar Pradesh), Utkal (Orissa), Marathwada (Maharashtra), Madhurai-Kamaraj (Tamil Nadu) and Banaras Hindu University offer Post Graduate and/or PhD courses in selected fisheries related subjects including aquaculture and marine sciences.

States such as Andhra Pradesh, Bihar, Haryana, Kerala, Karnataka, Maharashtra, Orissa and Tamil Nadu have introduced vocational courses in Aquaculture, Fishing Craft and Gear, Fisheries, Fish Processing, Inland Fisheries, Marine Fisheries and Maintenance and Repair of Marine Engines at 10 +2 level. ICAR fisheries institutes conduct short-term trainings of varying duration on various aspects of fisheries and aquaculture targeting fishers, entrepreneurs, scientists and teachers. The Freshwater Fish Farmers' Development Agency (FFDA) and Brackishwater Fish Farmers' Development Agency (BFDA) also undertake massive trainings in semi-intensive fish and prawn aquaculture. Private institutions like MAC School of Aquaculture, Toothukudi; Raman Academy, Kakkinada, etc. conduct

Diploma and PG Diploma course in Aquaculture and short-term trainings on various aspects of shrimp, prawn and fish farming.

Fisheries Management Information

The management regimes such as registration of fishing vessels, observation of closed fishing seasons, proscription of destructive fishing methods, implementation of mesh size regulations, reduction of by-catch and discards are concerned with the sustainable development of fisheries by establishing effective monitoring, control and surveillance in compliance with CCRF and other international rules and regulations. Information of these regimes is necessary for fisheries management. The important legal frameworks for fisheries management are listed below:

Central Legal Frameworks are:

- Comprehensive Marine Fishing Policy 2004.
- Guidelines for Fishing Operations in Indian EEZ.
- Letter of intent for operation of Fishing Vessels and
- The Draft Marine Fishing Regulation and Management Bill 2009

International obligations of India related to fisheries are:

- United Nations Convention on the Law of the Sea (UNCLOS).
- United Nations Fish Stock Agreement 1995 (UNFSA)
- Convention on Biological Diversity (CBD)
- Convention on International Trade in Endangered Species of Wild Fauna and Flora (CITES)
- Convention on Wetlands (RAMSAR)
- Convention on Migratory Species of Wild Animals (CMS), etc.

Fisheries Extension Information

The National Commission on Agriculture (1976) refers to extension as an informal, out-of-school education and services for the members of the farm family and others directly or indirectly engaged in farm production, to enable them to adopt improved practices in production, management, conservation and marketing (Sarkar *et al* 2007).

Agricultural Extension has been defined as 'a service or system which assists farm people through educational procedures in improving farming methods and techniques, increasing production efficiency and income, bettering their levels of living, and lifting the social and educational standards of rural life' (Maunder 1973). Carole and Stone (1989) opine that the primary purpose of aquaculture extension is to improve production of aquatic organisms for food and wealth for farmers, as well as for the nation as a whole.

Fisheries and aquaculture extension, as agricultural extension, is now recognized as a potent and critical force in the development process. Developmental institutions extension works comprise of demonstration of diversified fishing methods, popularization of diversified fishery products, periodical publication of resource survey results, etc. The extension activity under the State governments are oriented towards popularization of fish culture through supply of seed, training, nursery and pond management, improved methods of fishing techniques, fish handling and processing. Extension pamphlets, bulletins, handouts and posters on fishery themes, audio-visual publicity, organization/ participation in local/ national/ international workshops, fairs and exhibitions are the tools of extension activities.

The extension activities have unique problems in fisheries to tackle. The results of research and development become meaningful when the innovations reach the end users. Research, developmental and industrial activities for best use of the resources need a well planned system. The message of responsible fisheries and sustainable aquaculture are also to be percolated in the sector.

Invisible College

NGOs, Voluntary Agencies, Societies and Associations are the change agents providing information and independent advice, ideas and expertise, education, training and guidance for joint problem solving and decision-making, thus enhancing the people's ability to manage their own lives and resources. As they also take part in the fisheries co-management, share the responsibility for making decisions about the management of a fishery, FAO assign an important role to NGOs in implementation of CCRF (Carole and Stone 1989). The members consist of scientists, technologists, educationists, policy makers and other experts in the field. They act as Invisible College, information intermediaries and information source in the sector.

According to Dr Abdul Kalam (2012) former President of India, the development of the nation with more than 600000 villages in which about 750 million citizens live, can be achieved only when the economic, social and ecological empowerment is conducted in a mission mode manner for the entire rural area. This would require integrated mission with multiple stakeholders, with value added technology, with spirit of enterprise, with world-class products based on core competencies in the rural areas. In order to achieve this goal, the institutions in the sector should have back-up of information resources, services and professionals. The succeeding chapters aim to map fisheries and allied institutions established in the sector. Their functions, modes of information dissemination, role of library and information divisions, services offered to the grassroots, etc., will be appraised in the following chapters.

❑❑❑

Chapter-5

Fisheries Information Management in India

The present society is a networked society. It is more information dependent than all previous ones. Information is vital for an understanding of the current complex situations in every sphere of life, to discover new relationships and to respond effectively to the challenges. Unless relevant and timely information is distributed, quality of development in any sector including fisheries cannot be ensured. In the last five decades, a variety of institutions sprang up whose main stock in trade is knowledge and information. India has number of institutions located in different parts for generation, utilization and dissemination of information devoted to research, education and development in fisheries and allied areas.

There are seventeen national fisheries institutions functioning in the country under different subsectors of fisheries. These institutions are cited in Appendix 1. The overall aims and objectives of the library and information divisions in these institutions are based on the mission statement of the parent institutions. The functional phases of fisheries libraries are given in Table 5.

Table 5. Functional Phases of Fisheries Libraries

Stage	Objectives	Functions
1	To build up information resources	Acquisition; Storing; Cooperative agreements for resource sharing
2	To support education, research, extension and development	Acquisition; Storing; Organization; Mechanisms for sharing of information/ documents/ collections
3	To fulfill the information and the knowledge requirements of the users	Acquisition; Storing; Organization; Sharing; Information Services for categories of users such as Students,

		faculty, researchers, extension workers, decision makers, farmers, fishers and other stake holders
4	To continuously assess the information requirements	Surveys, user studies, Orientation on Collections; Organization; Information Services; Resource sharing mechanisms
5	To create necessary information bases	Cyclic from Stage 1 to 5, through Stage 4 for Traditional; Networked and Electronic sources of information.
6	To provide information support to the systems and all the user communities	Cyclic from Stage 1 to 5 by utilizing ICT enabled resources, media and services on need-based, locale-specific and demand-driven information.
7	To disseminate information without barriers of time, space, language etc to all the stakeholders	IM by initiating Global services on WWW, OPACs, ETDs, Repositories, Archives, Web Pages, Portals with multi-language operability.

Information support systems and services are shaped mainly by the research and development programmes, quality and quantum of scientific works, etc., carried out in the parent institutions. Information cycle operative in the sector is diagrammatically represented in Fig 1. In a typical university, library is one of the major statutory divisions headed by a statutory officer in second level of management with wide administrative and financial powers. Libraries have status equal to other academic and scientific divisions in SAUs and other educational institutions. In a typical ICAR institution, library comes at third or fourth level such as laboratories and other common facilities. Libraries are not represented in the national institutions namely FSI, NIFPHAAT, NFDB and CMLRE.

Library functions can generally be divided into a dozen distinguished functions. Mostly, only one professional is deployed in fisheries libraries. Exceptions are CMFRI and CIFT. In ICAR system, LIS professionals are engaged in routine works and managerial responsibilities are not assigned to them. Library and information systems under DAHDF are very limited. In general, library and information management and its applications are very feeble in the sector.

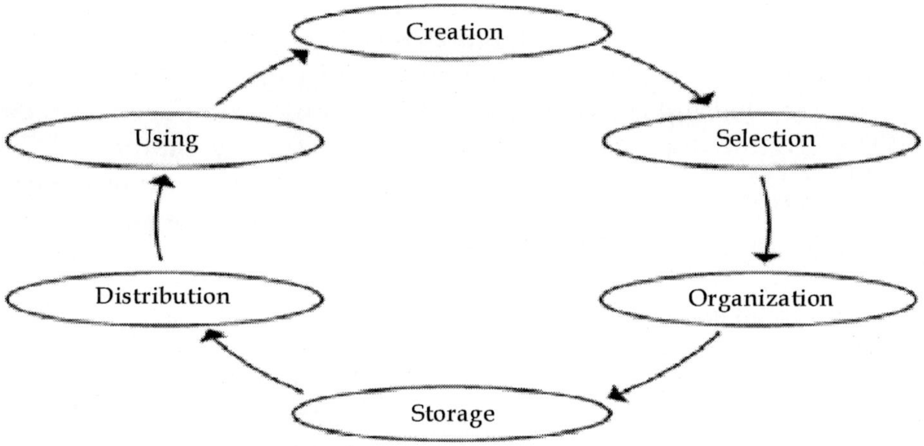

Figure 1. Fisheries Information Cycle

Libraries are the mechanisms that manage information and knowledge in the sector. They are fundamental to study, research and instruction in higher education. Traditional information services are searching and tracing, Current Awareness, Selective Dissemination of Information, abstracting and indexing, reference services, etc. The study evaluated some of the major aspects of library services, processes and activities that are easy to apply, relevant and reliable in order to find usefulness, effectiveness and inadequacies of fisheries information sector. Information services and products available in the sector are listed in Table 6.

Table 6. Information Services and Products in Fisheries Libraries

Services and Products	Institutions
Current Awareness	CIFRI, CIFE, CMFRI, CIFT, MPEDA
Bibliographies/ Indexing/ Abstracting	CIFRI (Fisheries Abstract) CMFRI (Bibliographies)
Literature Search	CMFRI, CIFT, MPEDA (on demand)
SDI	Nil
Publications	CIFRI (Fisheries Abstracts) CMFRI (CMFRI News letter)
Digital Archives/ Repositories	CMFRI (eprints@cmfri on OAI) CIFT (Digital Library@CIFT; in-house access) MPEDA (eprints@RGCA on OAI)

Library collections form the basic resources for providing various types of information services. Library collections are in various formats such as books, journals, theses, reports, microfiche, posters, maps, charts, etc. that are conventional. EIS constitute web pages, Portals, ETDs, Digital Repositories, Digital Archives, a-v materials, CD ROMSs/ Digital Video Discs (DVD), online databases, e-journals, e-books and such wide variety of materials. Major categories of fisheries information resources in libraries are given in Table 7.

Table 7. Categories of Resources in the Libraries

Print Documents	Electronic Information Sources
Books	e-Books
Journals	e-Journals
Back Volume	e-Journal archive/roll-back subscription
Theses/Dissertations	ETDs (In-house and OA)
Reports, reprints	Digital Repository/Archive/Library
A & I Services	Online Databases
Maps, Charts,Posters, etc.	Digital resources online/offline/OA/ Subscribed sources/Free Search
Reference/Statistics/Dictionaries	Online Reference/Statistical databases subscribed/Free access. Portals, Home pages

Fisheries Research System under ICAR has the largest number of scientists. CIFE has the biggest document resources. CIFE, CIFRI, CMFRI and CIFT have the largest collections in the sector. Document resource of the sector is satisfactory when taken in their whole but inadequate in the sub-systems when they are considered as separate compartments. There is also unnecessary duplication of resources. Survey to quantify the resources has excluded video tapes from audio-visual materials as they have only physical stock value in the libraries. These media are not supported by present day equipments/ technology. Book is taken as the representative sample for ascertaining strength of the documentary sources because of the accuracy of the data. Fourteen libraries had major collection of documents and five had less than 500 books in their collections. Strength of books in the libraries is presented in Figure 2.

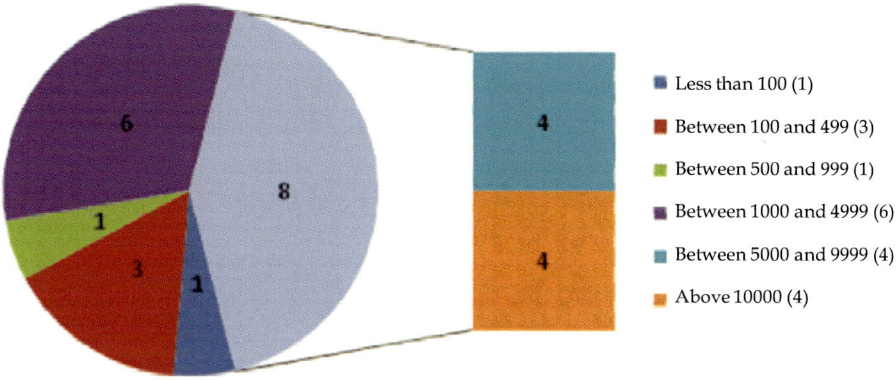

Figure 2. Strength of Books in the National Fisheries Libraries

The quantum of various subjects represented in the book collections of the national fisheries institutions are given in Fig 3. For the study, fisheries subjects were categorized into seven broad areas viz Aquatic Ecosystem and Fishery Environment; Aquatic Food Products and Technology; Aquaculture and Biotechnology; Fisheries Resource Management and Harvest Technology; Management and Social Sciences; Ocean Sciences, Technology and Engineering; and General and Miscellaneous. Collections on Aquatic Ecosystem and Fishery Environment (AE&FE) constitutes 13%; Aquatic Food Products and Technology (AFP&T) constitutes 13%; Aquaculture and Biotechnology (Aq&BT) 9%; Fisheries Resource Management and Harvest Technology (FRM&HT) 17%; Management and Social Sciences (M&SS) 18%; Ocean Sciences, Technology and Engineering (OSTE) 8%; and General and Miscellaneous (Gen& Misc) constitutes 22% of the total collections in the sector.

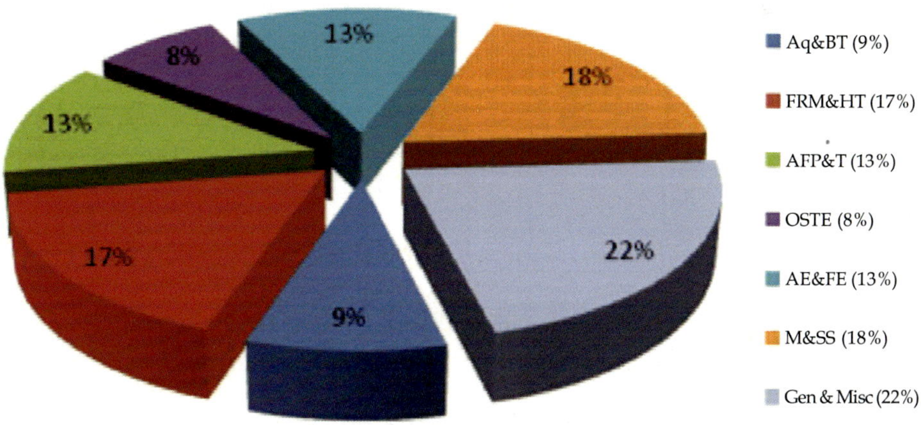

Figure 3. Subject Representation in Book Collection

Electronic Information Sources (EIS) is a major resource in modern libraries. CIFNET, NIFPHATT, FSI, CICEF, NFDB, CAA, CMLRE and FISHCOPFED did not hold any EIS. CMFRI is the only institution that hosted Digital Archive on Open Access. Though the international publishers, mainly Wiley, Teylor & Francis, Academic Press, CABI and EBC publish approximately 500 books on fisheries subjects which also have e-version, subscription of e-books are not common in the sector. It seems that the fisheries sector lacks awareness about usage of EIS. Familiarization/sensitization programmes may catalyze use of e-resources in the sector. ASFA is the major database subscribed in National fisheries institutions. However, resource sharing and cooperation for maximum utilization of such databases are absent.

National fisheries institutions subscribe to a number of international journals. They also use CeRA resources (CeRA is explained in Chapter 8, under heading Initiatives of ICAR) which include subscribed journals as well as the Open Access e-journals. Nevertheless, the fisheries institutions duplicate a number of foreign journals in addition to its availability in the sector or in CeRA at a huge cost. The list of journals duplicated in addition to their access in CeRA is given in Table 8.

Table 8. Foreign Journals Duplicated in Central Fisheries Institutions in addition to CeRA

S. No.	Journals included in CeRA	Price	No. of Inst. duplicated journals	Total Cost
1	Agricultural Information Worldwide	5979	1	5979
2	Aquaculture	241076	7	1687532
3	Aquaculture Asia Pacific	3500	1	3500
4	Aquaculture Economics and Management	24148	3	72444
5	Aquaculture International	76329	4	305316
6	Aquatic Ecosystem and Health Management	27434	2	54868
7	Fish and Shellfish Immunology	45978	5	229890
8	Fish Physiology and Biochemistry	47862	4	191448
9	Fisheries Research	126084	3	378252
10	Fishery Bulletin	2383	1	2383
11	Global Aquaculture Advocate	5624	2	11248

12	Hydrobiologia	912240	2	1824480
13	Journal of Applied Aquaculture	26440	4	105760
14	Marine Pollution Bulletin	86125	2	172250
15	National Geographic	1702	1	1702
16	Reviews in Fisheries Science	55341	3	166023
	Total	1688245	45	5213075

Duplication in subscriptions results in loss of foreign exchange. There were 48 costly journals duplicated in the sector. Eleven foreign journals were found to be subscribed by more than five institutions. There were 117 duplications in foreign journals in total and 16 foreign journals were found duplicated by fisheries institutions in addition to its availability in CeRA. The foreign journals subscribed by CMFRI are also available in CSIR e-journal Consortium viz., National Knowledge Resource Consortium (NKRC). Twenty four online journals subscribed by CMFRI are seen available in CSIR Consortium. NIO Kochi campus is only few yards away from CMFRI HQs.

The amount spent on journals has not shown any sign of reduction though CeRA subscribes to a number of international journals in fisheries and related subjects. The possible reasons for this situation are (1) escalation in price of International journals (2) important fisheries journals are not included in CeRA (3) subscription in addition to the availability in CeRA. Whatever, duplicating the journals in addition to CeRA is unjustifiable at all costs. Resource sharing and cooperation among intra and inter organizations are absent in the sector. Formulation of minimum norms for cooperation shall save our exchequer with crores of Indian money.

Finance is important and necessary for library and information services as water for fish. Agricultural University Library Commission (1967) recommends for at least 6% of the total operating budget of an institution towards library allocations. Figure 4 compares institutional budget against budget allotments for libraries in the national fisheries institutions for five years from 2006-07 to 2010-11. It is noted that the budgetary allocations fluctuate from year to year and there is no definite pattern followed for allocations.

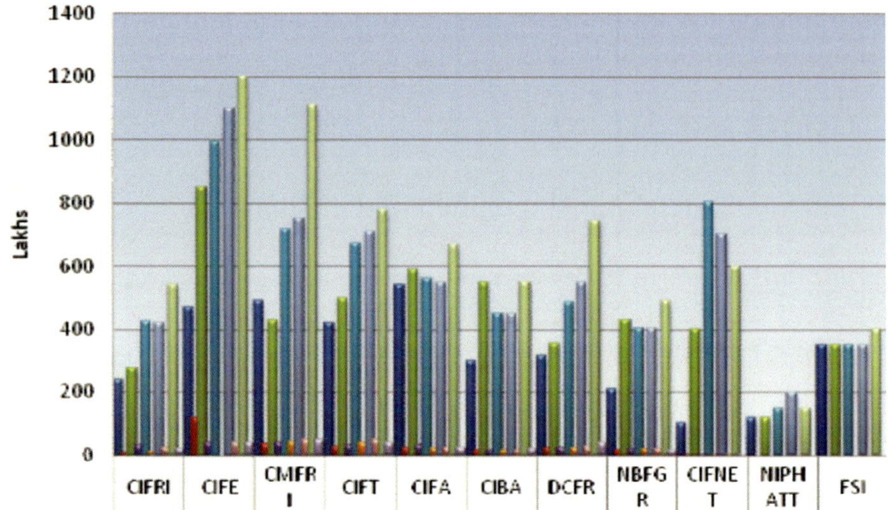

	CIFRI	CIFE	CMFRI	CIFT	CIFA	CIBA	DCFR	NBFGR	CIFNET	NIPHATT	FSI
2006-07 IB	240	469	493	420	540	300	317	209	102	120	350
2006-07 LB	9	121	35.5	30	25	15	25	15	3	0	0
2007-08 IB	278	850	429	500	592	548	354	430	400	120	350
2007-08 LB	31	40	40	35	35	15	25	20	4	0	0
2008-09 IB	425	995	720	675	560	450	487	405	804	150	349
2008-09 LB	11	0	45	40	25	15	25	20	3	0	0
2009-10 IB	420	1100	750	710	550	450	550	405	700	200	350
2009-10 LB	23	40	50	50	25	15	28	20	3	0	0
2010-11 IB	540	1200	1109	780	670	550	744	490	600	150	400
2010-11 LB	21	40	50	40	25	21	40	18	2	0	0

Figure 4. Institutional vs Library Budget of National Fisheries Institutions

Comparison of library budget of the national fisheries institutions for five years from 2006-07 to 2010-11 is given in Figure 5. There is no progressive pattern indicating increase in the library allocation except CMFRI and CIFT. CMFRI had same allocation as of the previous year in 2010-11 whereas CIFT had a fall in allocation. CIFNET under DAHDF shows progressive fall in the allocations whereas other two institutions viz., NIPHATT and FSI had no allocations for library at all.

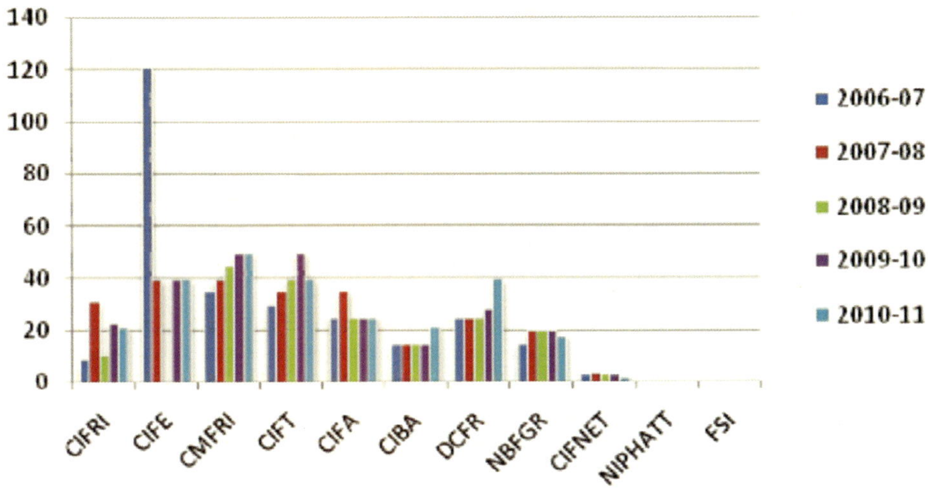

Figure 5. Library Budget of National Fisheries Institutions

Figure 6 shows the amount spent on journals in the national fisheries institutions for the last five years. Figure 7 shows the amount spent on books in the national fisheries institutions for the last five years. It is seen that National fisheries research institutions maintain titles of Indian and International Journals uniformly over the years. They spend about 75-80% of library budget for journals every year leaving behind small amounts for purchase of books.

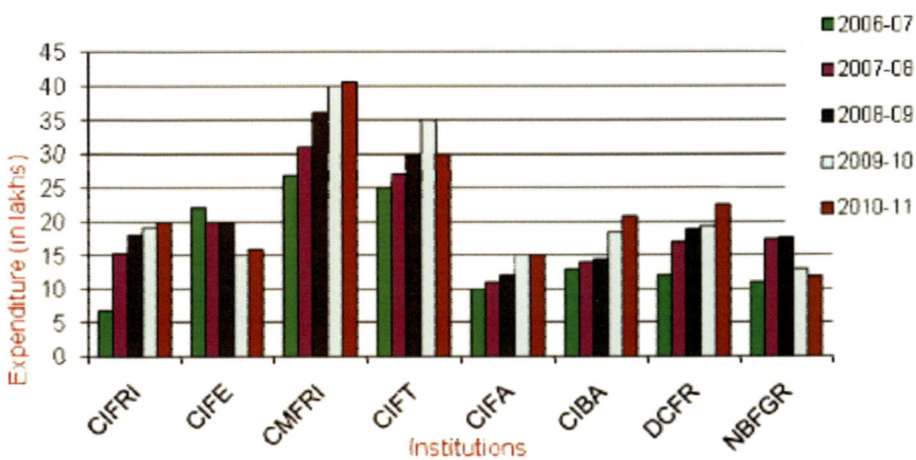

Figure 6. Expenditure on Journals in National Fisheries Institutions

Costs of publications are escalating. New and interdisciplinary subjects and publications are also on the rise. Institutions are unable to maintain the pace of literature output in the field. Therefore, subject specialized collections in each sub-system of fisheries need to be developed so that these libraries can function as specialized Information Centres and gateways in that particular sub-system. Presently, the collection development is haphazard and no thought of specialization is given in the sector. Cost-effectiveness is not made the riding principle for collection development.

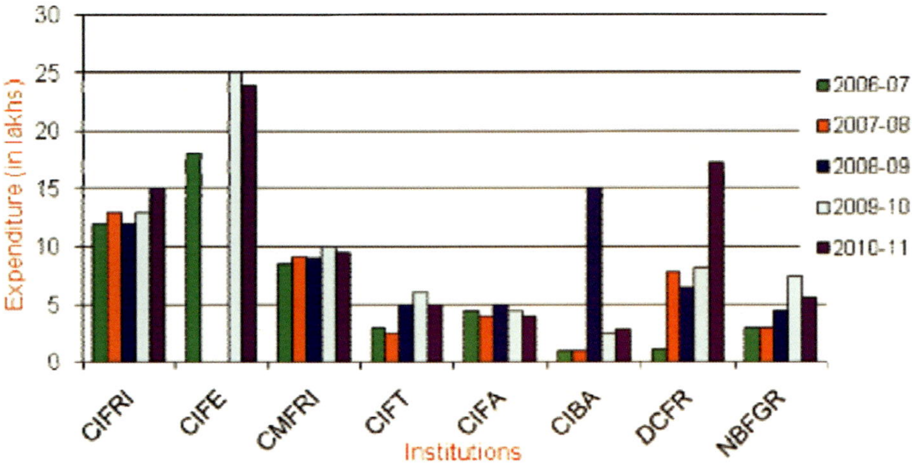

Figure 7. Expenditure on Books in National Fisheries Institutions

Fisheries is a multi disciplinary subject. It draws theoretical base from basic sciences. Economics, Statistics, Management, Aquatic; Environment; Physical; Live and Engineering Sciences and Technology subjects nurture it. Academic institutions may have to build collections accordingly. Research institutions, however can narrow the collections to the core and specialization achieved by them.

Fisheries Educational Institutions

Professional fisheries education for the managerial and technical categories of personnel are imparted through the graduate and post-graduate level courses at the Central/ State Agricultural/ Veterinary/ Fisheries Universities. Besides Fisheries Colleges, a number of institutions offer fisheries related courses. Altogether, a strong network of fisheries educational institutions could be formed, spreading throughout the length and breadth of India. Entire North-Eastern states are covered under Central Agricultural University, Imphal for education in fisheries science. List of fisheries universities/colleges in India is given in Appendix 2, Section A and Specialized courses offered by them in Section B. Strength of documents in the colleges is given in Figure 8.

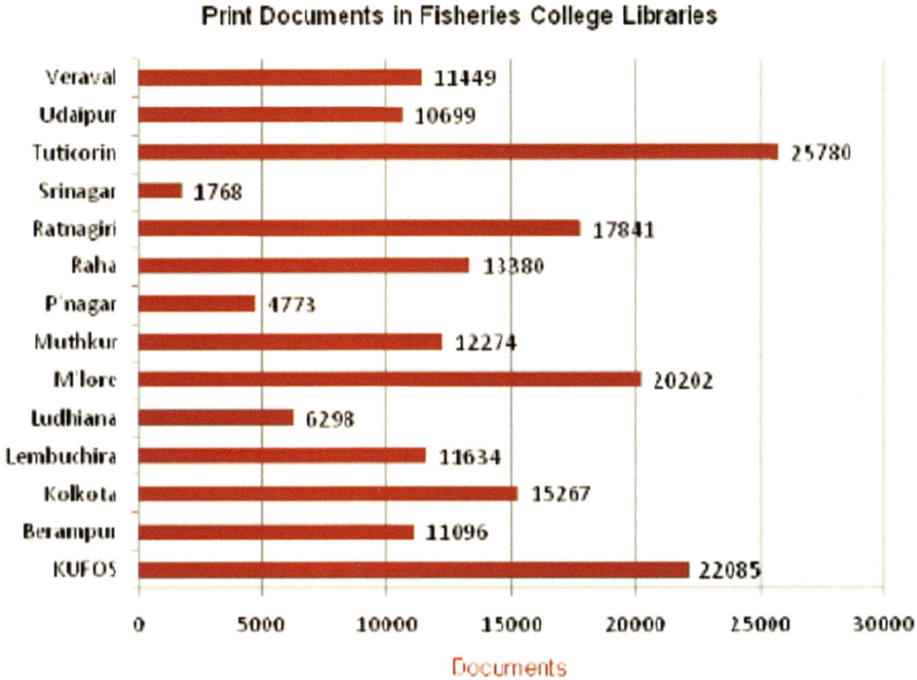

Figure 8. Print Documents in Fisheries College Libraries

Fisheries colleges have good strength of print documents. The major holders are FCRI, Tuticorin; KUFOS, Kochi and CoF, Mangalore. CoF Srinagar is a nascent one. Resources of CoF Pantnagar are pooled with Central Library, GBPUAT.

As per the survey results, fisheries universities/colleges have access to top line services (international and national). SAUs and Fisheries colleges under ICAR have access to CeRA services. CoF Pantnagar has the advantage of access to CSIR and UGC networks as the resources are pooled in Central Library, GBPUAT. Although ASFA is the main bibliographic database in fisheries, all the colleges were not subscribing it. Resource sharing in the sub-regions of the country can provide better opportunity for access to costly databases by the students and teachers. Table 9 gives details of top line information services available in fisheries college libraries.

Table 9. Online Information Services Available in Fisheries Colleges

Top Line Services	Institution	Access
ICAR Network (CeRA)	All fisheries universities/colleges	Static IP Based. Free access for ICAR/SAUs
UGC Network	CoF, Pantnagar	Central Library, GBPUAT (Pooled Resources)
CSIR Network	CoF, Pantnagar	Central Library, GBPUAT (Pooled Resources)
ASFA database	KUFOS; CoF Raha, Mang'lr, Tuticorin and Kolkata	Subscription. Static IP based access
CABI/Wiley/etc Databases/e-Book	Nil	
FAO Information services/flagship publications	All	OA
IndiaStat.com	CoF Pantnagar & Raha	Subscription

In the fisheries education sub-system, there are two streams, one under the ICAR/SAUs and the other under UGC catering to the professional needs of the sector. The quantum of document collection under these streams is significant. The major source of finance for colleges and universities is ICAR aid. Colleges have good collection of books but weak journal collections. CeRA forms the major EIS for the sector. However, use of EIS is not frequent and quantum of subscription of e-books, online databases and e-journals is low in the sector. Resource wise, libraries under ICAR and fisheries college libraries are in a comfortable zone.

Major Out-stream Institutions

Various institutions outside fisheries sector are engaged in problem-oriented research on planning, management, production, processing, marketing, input supply systems, agricultural finance, social change in rural areas, socio-economic development of rural poor and other areas related to fisheries. These institutions form Major Out-stream Institutions in view of their importance for fisheries sector and are listed in Appendix 3. Section A of Appendix 3 lists institutions; Section B lists Programmes, NGOs and Associations of national standing, Section C lists Organizations for aquatic environment protection, coastal management, etc. and in Section D, Learned societies fostering Fisheries and allied sciences by publishing/ conducting scholarly journals, handbooks, manuals, seminars, symposia, workshops *etc.* are given.

Fishery Sector Institutional Finance

There exists an elaborate structure of institutional finance which could cater to the growing requirements of the fisheries sector. The major sources of long-term finance for capital expenditure are various term lending institutions such as Industrial Finance Corporation of India (IFCI), Industrial Credit and Investment Corporation of India (ICICI) and Industrial Development Bank of India (IDBI). These institutions provide financial support either directly through their specialized subsidiaries to deal with specific sectors such as Shipping Credit and Investment Corporation of India (SCICI) or through the State Finance Corporations (SFC) (Srivastava et al 1991).

The National Bank for Agriculture and Rural development (NABARD) also operates as a separate financial agency to provide refinancing facility for the primary lending to agricultural and agro-industrial projects made by the commercial banks. All these finance institutions have good infrastructure, facilities and library resources. Currently, Shipping Credit and Investment Corporation of India (SCICI); Industrial Development Bank of India (IDBI); National Bank for Agriculture and Rural development (NABARD); and National Cooperative Development Corporation(NCDC), New Delhi are engaged in providing direct or indirect finance for the fisheries sector. NFDB and FISHCOPFED are the two different agencies for the development of the fisheries sector. NCDC has started promoting and developing fishery cooperatives after amendment of its Act in 1974 to cover fisheries within its purview.

Need for Resource Sharing and Consortium Activities in Fisheries Sector

The diversity of institutions, research and development activities, technological advancements, etc., underscores the need for the resource sharing, cooperation and collaborative research for the development of the sector. Analysis of the resources available in the libraries of fisheries institutions revealed that the resources taken together are significant for fisheries sector as a whole but not sufficient when individual libraries are considered as separate entities. Interlibrary lending and cooperative collection development are absent in the sector. Willingness, the economic imperatives, formal and informal agreements, etc., are to be evolved for resource sharing in the sector. ICT is another utility to endorse cooperative endeavors in the sector.

The institutional activities range from the broad to the narrow fields of specializations in the sector. Information resources in the fisheries institutions represent the information and knowledge repository of the sector. Presently, fisheries is abound with various issues such as environmental protection, sustainability issues in marine as well as inland fisheries, profitability of farm enterprises, women empowerment, rural development, liberalization and globalization processes under WTO regime, etc. The challenges posed by these factors call for better management of information and knowledge in the sector.

Consortium Research needs to be initiated in the sector by cluster institutions to solve umpteen issues by utilizing information resources in the sector. Inter-institutional participation and Consortium Research is the *manthra* for development of any sector. Agencies such as ICAR, SAUs, CSIR and DST engaged in fisheries and allied research are to be coordinated through strong cross-institutional interaction and robust information sharing and services for the development of fisheries sector. Fisheries science being a specialized branch of professional science involving aquatic science, marine science, ecology, environmental science, management science, etc., networking of the institutions involved in R&D, Education and Training is essential for fisheries development in the country.

The lack of information resource sharing in the sector is conspicuous. It is reflected even in subscribing foreign journals within ICAR System. Many of its fisheries institutions subscribe to the one and same costly foreign journals that is available either in CeRA or other subscription institutes. This indicates disregard to resource sharing, cost effectiveness and loss of public money. There is also no effective inter and intra mechanism for sharing fisheries related information resources among the main-stream and out-stream institutions in the country. The use and accessibility of costly resources and databases subscribed by various institutions in the sector are confined to the four walls of the national institutions. As information resource sharing is not evolved in the sector, exchange of information and exploration of ideas are not adequately utilized. Institutional memberships to IAMSLIC, Aquatic Commons, JSTOR, etc. that promote resource sharing are poor. Fisheries institutions need to partake in such global resource sharing programmes.

In general, fisheries libraries are passive towards networking, resource sharing, digitization, and informatics led services. Lack of policies, procedures, strategies, management initiatives, low awareness of higher officials and policy makers on ICT, etc., are the factors for this situation. These are coupled with the lack of qualified and experienced Library and Information Science professionals. Their status and pay scales are not at par with academic and scientific staff in fisheries institutions. UGC/ICAR prescribes norms, qualifications, selection and appointment for Librarians in higher education and research system. Nevertheless, ICAR itself is not following these norms in the education and research institutes under ICAR. CIFE, the Deemed University under ICAR, does not have University Librarian/ Deputy Librarian/ Assistant Librarian or equivalent. Libraries are only at fourth level in ICAR institutions like any common facility such as laboratory, canteen, etc. Head of the Library used to be a Division Head, a typical remote control operation. Another example, one of the oldest fisheries colleges in India does not have a College Librarian and qualified professionals for the last two decades. One English teacher designated as College Librarian, one professional on contract basis and one helper run the show there.

There are wide variations in the designations, scale of pay, qualifications and above all, apathy towards library and professionals in the sector as a whole. The role of libraries in fisheries information transfer is not adequately acknowledged and there are no significant roles given to libraries or library professionals in the programmes on documentation, information dissemination, as well as development of related products and services in the sector, especially in ICAR system.

❑❑❑

Chapter-6

Fisheries Information Resources and Services in Kerala

The State of Kerala was formed in 1956 as part of the linguistic re-organization of the Indian States by merging the three Malayalam speaking regions - the princely states of Travancore and Cochin and the Malabar district of the Madras Presidency. Its land area is 38,863 sq. km, stretching 580 km in length and 30-130 km in breadth. While in terms of area, Kerala forms only 1.1% of India, its population (in 2001) of 31.8 million accounts for 3.01% of India's. Population density in Kerala is 819 persons per sq. km, one of the highest in the country, often camouflaged by biotic green. Moreover, the population is spread across the State and there are no big urban agglomerations. Kochi (Cochin), the biggest city of Kerala, has a population of only about 0.27 million.

Kerala has three predominant religions. Christians and Muslims account for a greater share than seen in other Indian States and even all-India. In the 2011 census, they accounted for 18.38% and 26.56% of the population, respectively, with the Hindus mostly contributing the rest (54.72%). Ecology plays an important role in the Kerala economy. The diversified natural resource base enables a large degree of occupational diversification. Geographically, the region comprises three zones - low land, midland and high ranges. The low land, where the population density is the highest, consists of sandy and fertile soils of the river valleys, lakes and backwaters, providing the basis for fishing, rice and coconut cultivation and horticulture. Coconut, rice, cassava, arecanut and cashew, along with rubber, pepper, and ginger on the slopes pre-dominate the midland region. The high ranges, where the population density is the lowest, consist of natural evergreen tropical forests giving way to plantations of tea, coffee and rubber (Raman Nair 2004).

A striking feature of Kerala's development experience is the growth of the service sector. Historically too, this sector has been more pronounced in Kerala than in the rest of the country. The largest shares of income (55%) and employment (40%) are generated in the service sector. Kerala's economy is no longer predominantly agrarian; the primary sector accounts for only 26% of the State income and 32% of employment (as in 1999-2000). Kerala has an active political society compared to the rest of India. There is a high degree of political activism, the consequences of which are subject to differences of opinion. No single party has been able to form a Government of its own since the formation of Kerala. Currently, two coalitions have been ruling the State; neither of them having managed to win a consecutive term. While one is led by the Indian National Congress, the other is led by the Communist Party of India (Marxist). There are also parties that do not belong to either of the two coalitions, but these are yet to gain any electoral representation in the State Assembly (Oommen 1999).

Fisheries Sector of Kerala State

The three estate of the fishery economy viz., the water resources, the fish resources and the human resources are at a comfortable level in Kerala. Situated in the Southwest part of India, Kerala has a slender stretch of land with a long surf beaten coast on the western side and a lush green mountain range on the eastern side. The state has a coastline of 590 km and the EEZ extends up to 200 nautical miles far beyond the continental shelf, which covers an area of 218536 sq km providing opportunities in traditional fishing in inshore waters from ages. The inland sector is endowed with extensive inter-connected brackish water lakes and estuaries with a total area of 1,26,366 ha. Forty one west flowing and three east flowing rivers have a total length of 320 km and water spread area of 85000 ha. Reservoirs and minor irrigation tanks constitute 45725 ha. Tanks and Ponds have an area of 24310 ha (Government of Kerala 2010A). Technological interventions such as mechanization in the 1950s and the motorization in the 1980s caused several changes in fishing methods along the Kerala coast. The mechanized sector plays an important role in the fishery of Kerala contributing to about 66 per cent followed by the motorized sector contributing 27 per cent and the artisanal sector contributing 7 per cent. The inshore waters are under heavy or excessive fishing pressures and most of the resources are exploited optimally (Joice et al 2010). Fisherman population is 11.36 lakh, which include 8.28 lakh in marine and 3.28 lakh in inland sector. Active fishermen are estimated at 2.3 lakh. (1.8 marine and 0.5 lakh in inland sector) Fishermen settlement areas spread over 222 fishing villages in marine sector and 113 villages in inland sector (Government of Kerala 2009).

State's Fishing Community

Kerala boasts of the highest quality of life in the country as measured by human development indicators. However, the State's fishing community has largely been left out of the general development experience. Traditional fisher folk who had no other employment option suffered and as a community they continued to lag behind the rest of the State in all areas of development. Several factors such as low social status, poor economic conditions, illiteracy, leaning on middle-men, traditional fishing equipments and methods of fishing, low production rate and income influence the socio-economic conditions of fishermen. For the proper development of the fishing industry, socio-economic advancement of fishermen is considered essential not in Kerala alone but entire nation.

Department of Fisheries, Government of Kerala

Governance of the Fisheries sector is vested with the Minister for Fisheries. All the development and management programmes envisaged by the Government for the fisheries sector are implemented by the State Department of Fisheries. The chief executive responsible for fisheries in the government is the Secretary to the Government (Fisheries). The Department of Fisheries, headed by the Director of Fisheries, is structurally stratified and organized under state (Director of Fisheries), zonal (Joint Directors of South, Central and North zone), district (Deputy Directors) and panchayat (Fisheries Sub Inspectors in *Matsyabhavans*) levels. Agencies viz., Matsyafed, ADAK, KFWEB, FIRMA and FFDA implement the Government's visions and schemes in the sector (Government of Kerala 2012; 2013).

The government and Fisheries Department have various projects and programs for increasing production, for conserving and ensuring sustainable exploitation of fisheries wealth, for promoting cultivation of fish and prawns, for development of fishing harbours, for strengthening facilities for landing of fish, for strengthening facilities for marketing of fish, and for the up-lift and welfare of the fisher folk.

Way back in 1988, Kerala set the trend in using an annual fishing closure as a tool in the management of fisheries resources, and several coastal States in India have subsequently followed this route. Ban on monsoon trawling has proved to be an effective measure to conserve the fishery resources for the sustainable development of the fishery in the state (Government of Kerala 2011).

Matsya Bhavans in 200 Panchayats act as the field offices of the Department of Fisheries, linking to the grass roots of the sector. Department and its agencies maintain hatcheries at Neyyar Dam, Neendakara, Pannivelichira, Polachira, Pallam, Azheecode, Malampuzha, Odayam (ADAK), and Wynad (FIRMA) (Government of Kerala 2010B). Hatcheries serve the farmers with quality seeds. The system of official statistics in the State of Kerala is decentralized. Directorate of Economics and Statistics (DES) is responsible for collection, compilation and dissemination of statistics on all socio-economic aspects of the State. As Line Departments are responsible for statistical activities, Fisheries Statistics are generated by Fisheries Department (Government of India, 2010). A discussion on the Government agencies playing direct roles in implementing programmes for the socio-economic development of the rural poor in the sector are given in Appendix 4, Section A.

Universities and Colleges Offering Fisheries Courses

Universities, Colleges and other affiliated institutions offering various courses in fisheries and related subjects cater to the needs of human resources, skills and technology required for the sustainable development of fisheries sector in the State. These institutions have information resources on fisheries, fish farming and socio-economic aspects related to fisheries sector in English as well as in Malayalam. Universities, Schools and Colleges that offer fisheries courses are given in Appendix 4, Section B.

Out-stream Institutions of Kerala State

Institutions engaged in implementation of programmes for the socio-economic development of the rural poor in the State having direct or indirect roles with the fisheries sector are discussed in the following sections. These institutions have information resources mainly on socio-economic topics related to fisheries sector. However, utilization of these resources is not spread in the sector due to absence of resource sharing mechanisms. Out stream institutions, bigger and smaller, of Kerala state is given as Appendix 4, Section C. The NGOs, Voluntary organizations, Societies operating in the State of Kerala are given in Appendix 4, Section D.

Information Resources in Fisheries and Allied Institutions

The State of Kerala has large number of institutions for generation, utilization and dissemination of information devoted to research, education and development in fisheries and allied areas under various organizational streams. In all these institutions, library/ documentation/information centres are the functional base for information resources and services to its clientele. The resources mainly constitute the conventional sources such as books, journals, theses, reports, etc. Electronic Information Sources (EIS) such as web, Portals, Electronic Thesis and Dissertations (ETDs), Digital Repositories, Digital Archives, audio-visual materials, CDs/DVDs, online databases, e-journals, e-books, etc. also made entry into the libraries in the sector. Resources in the institutions situated in Kerala State are discussed in the following sections. Figure 9 presents strength of print documents in education institutions.

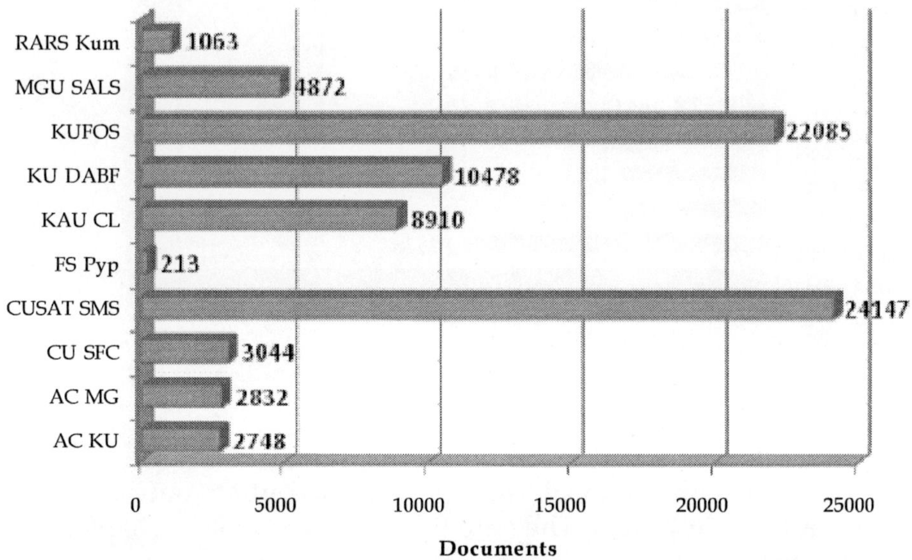

Figure 9. Print Documents in Fisheries Education Institution libraries in Kerala

Figure 10 presents strength of print resources in other fisheries institutions. When print documents in fisheries education institutional libraries in Kerala is considered, School of Marine Sciences Library, CUSAT tops the list followed by KUFOS; Centre of Advanced Study in Aquatic Biology and Fisheries, Kerala University; and Central Library, Kerala Agricultural University. NIO Regional Centre, Kochi; Regional Centres of CMFRI; SALS, MG University; Regional Centre, ZSI; and CFS, Trivandrum also have good number of resources.

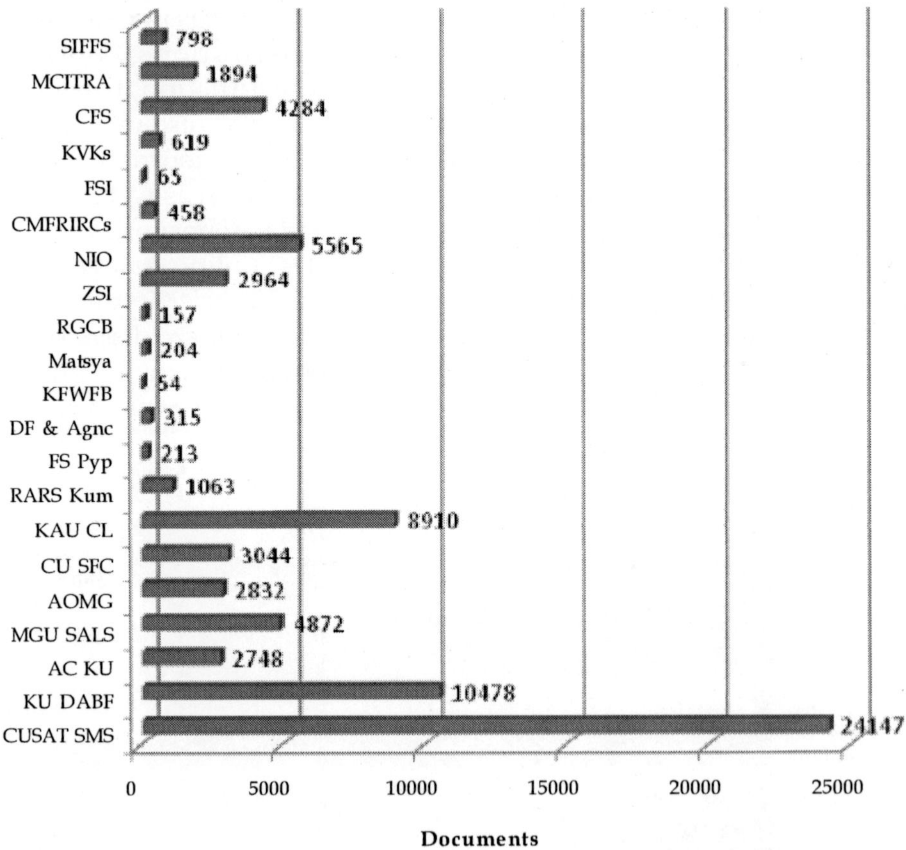

Figure 10. Print Documents in Fisheries Institution Libraries in Kerala

There are many national fisheries as well as out-stream institutions headquartered in Kerala. They are dealt in the previous chapter. The national fisheries as well as out-stream institutions have a number of Regional Centres and they have considerable quantum of fisheries information resources. Regional / Zonal Centres of Central Fisheries Institutions and other Out-stream Institutions situated in Kerala State viz., (1) CMFRI: Kozhikode, Vizhinjam, Njnarakkal (KVK), Quilon. (2) FSI: Kochi (3) MPEDA: Kochi, Njnarakkal, Vizhinjam (RGCB). (4) ZSI: Kozhikode (5) CIFRI: Kochi (6) NBFGR: Kochi (7) NIO: Kochi and (8) EIA: Kochi. Figure 11 presents strength of print documents in the Regional Centres of National Fisheries and allied Institutions situated in Kerala. Among Regional Centres, NIO Kochi has rich resources followed by ZSI, Kozhikode. Kochi Regional Centres of CIFRI and NBFGR are housed in CMFRI HQs, Kochi and utilize its resources.

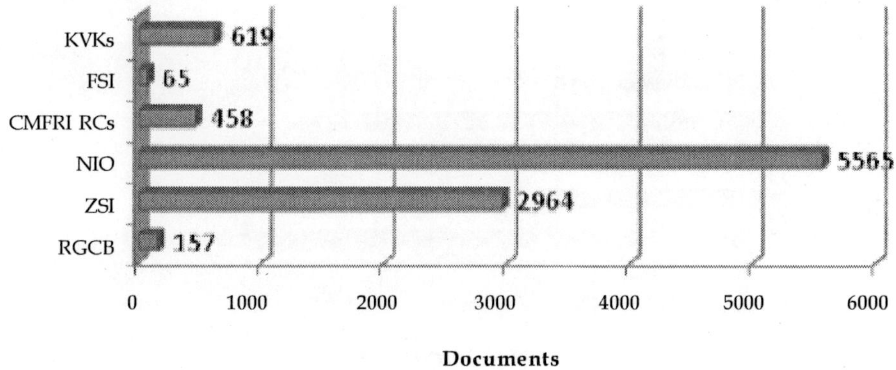

Figure 11. Print Documents in the Regional Centres of Central Institutions in Kerala

There are institutions, big and small, directly or indirectly related to the fisheries sector in Kerala, varying from institutions of international standing such as CDS and KFRI, institutions of national standing such as SIRD, CESS (presently National Centre for Earth Sciences Studies) and CWRDM to small establishment like State Resource Centre-Kerala (SRC-K). Figure 12 presents strength of print documents in out stream institution libraries in Kerala.

CDS has biggest collection, followed by KFRI, CESS, CWRDM and SIRD. The resources are mainly on socio-economic, socio-cultural, ecological, extension, earth and water studies. CFRD, KIED, KREWS and SRC have very limited resources. Matsyafed, ADAK, KFWEB, FIRMA and FFDA, the implementing agencies of the government programmes generally do not have any information resources and services to serve on farming, technology updates, etc in English as well as in the regional language. The staff acts as the information link between the agency and the fishers/fish farmers in the sector. Implementation of State's schemes depends on the budgetary provisions and funds available. There are number of government agencies with overlapping aims and objectives. This makes the stakeholders running from pillar to post enquiring about schemes, technical advice, etc. Amalgamation/ liquidation/ reduction of these agencies by the government shall save the stakeholders as well as public money.

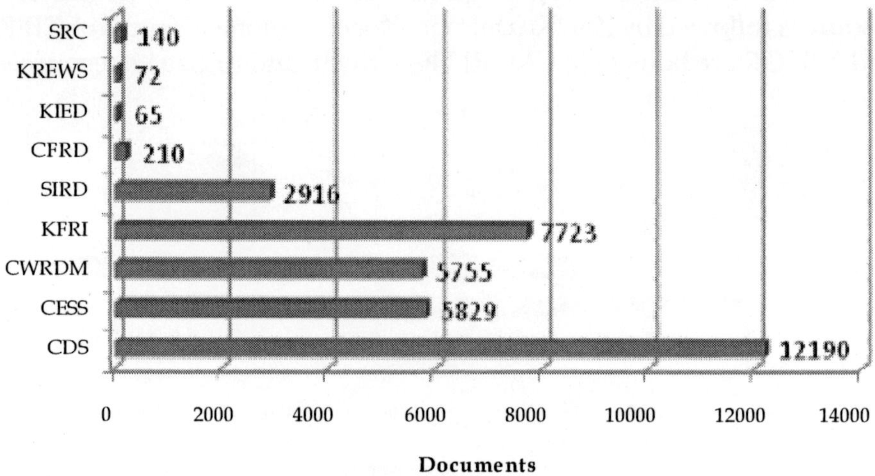

Figure 12. Print Documents in the Out-steam Institution Libraries in Kerala

The NGOs, Voluntary organizations, Societies operating in the State of Kerala have significant information resources on fisheries communities, socio-economic-cultural studies, etc. The approach of these agencies is small-scale and their activity is oriented to the grass-roots. Information resources of these agencies were also the subject of study. Figure 13 presents the consolidated strength of resources in the major fisheries institution libraries in Kerala including that of Centre for Fisheries Studies (NGO).

The strength of resources varies from institution to institution. Fisheries educational institution libraries have good resources where as Department of Fisheries and agencies under it do have neither library system nor information services. Document sources in Regional Centres of central institutions viz., NIO and ZSI are good. NGOs have libraries with organized collections. It is found that the CDS, CESS *(Now NCESS)*, CWRDM, KFRI and SIRD have good strength of print documents in fisheries and related subjects. The State government institutions have very weak information resources.

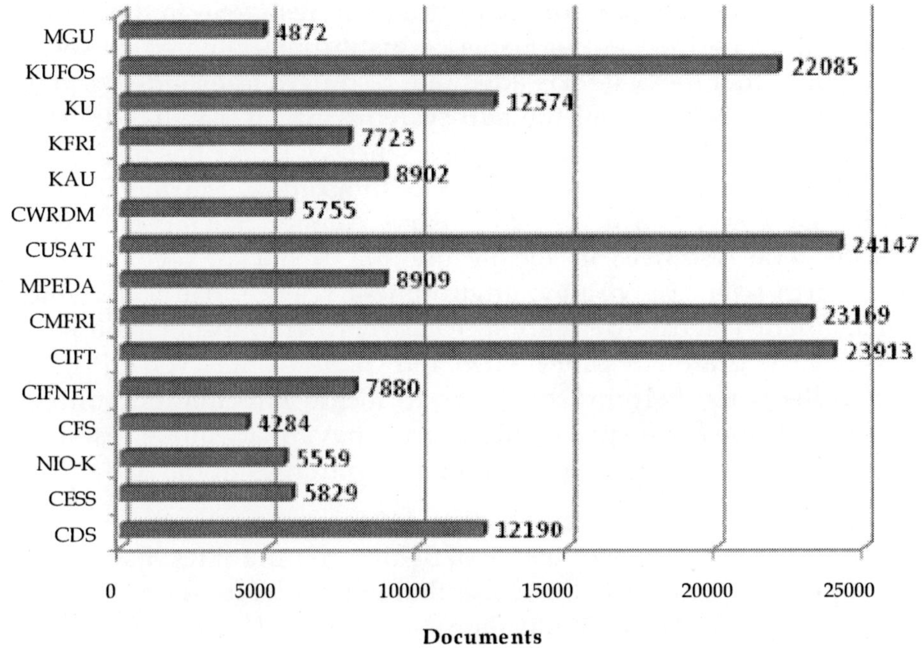

Figure 13. Resources in the Major Institutions in Kerala

Kochi region has high concentration of fisheries institutions and therefore, the region has the resources to function as fisheries information hub for the country and has the capacity to emerge as the Fisheries Knowledge Hub of the country. Figure 14 presents print document resources in the Kochi Region. Kochi region has the information potential to emerge as Fisheries Knowledge City, supported and funded by visionary programmes of the Governments.

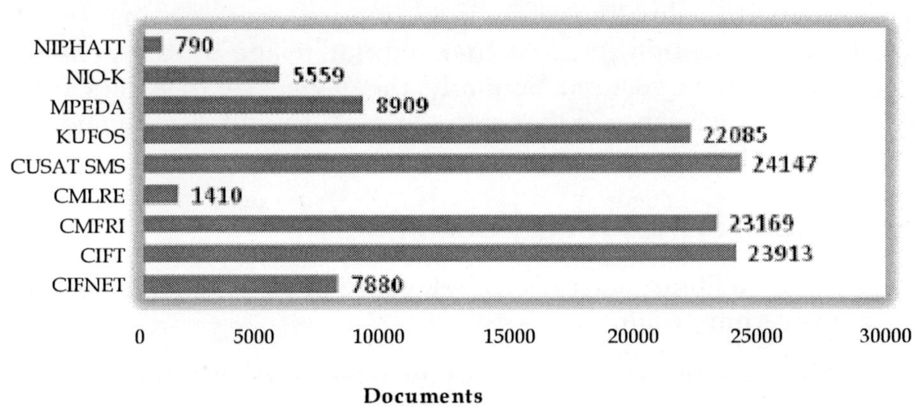

Figure 14. Print Document Resources in the Kochi Region

Considering the quantum of information resources in the State of Kerala including the Central Fisheries Institutions situated in Kerala, it is evident that the State has adequate resources in fisheries, aquatic and related subjects in all the sub-systems viz., research, education and extension. The School of Marine Sciences, CUSAT has the highest strength of documents, including Oceanography, Marine Biology, Marine Geology, Marine Geochemistry, Aquatic Science and allied subjects. The resources in socio-economic, financial, socio-cultural, rural, earth sciences, ecology, environment science, nautical science, management, extension, etc. are spread over to a number of institutions in Kerala. At present, CMFRI, CDS and CUSAT offer Web OPAC on their collections, helping the users to locate information sources. However, Fisheries institutional libraries have inadequate resources for neo-literates, farming and fishing communities in the State.

Non-governmental and non-profit organizations generate information for the developments of fishing communities. Pamphlets, mails, print news, etc. are the dissemination media for them. *Samudra* (English) of ICSF, *Alakal* (Malayalam) of Kerala Federation of Fisheries Workers are some of the newsletters in the sector. National and local dailies disseminate information on habitat destruction, over fishing, harmful chemicals, seafood toxicity, etc. NGOs have significant collection of fisheries documents in regional languages.

Computer awareness, facilities and access points are to be spread to the grass-roots to enable information access and dissemination. Computer facilities in the village schools may be tuned to function as VKC/VIC/Internet Centre also for the benefit of primary stakeholders in fisheries sector. These centres should adequately provide a host of services on rural livelihood such as finance, markets, insurance, healthcare, education, etc., so that regular usage by the primary stakeholders can be ensured. Similarly, the *Akshaya* centres, the service points for e-Governance in the State of Kerala should also function as VKC/VIC in fishing villages.

Perceptions of the Primary Stakeholders

Studies on library user needs, relevance of information available, etc. are very important:

- To improve the user experience and make the resources key to their needs

- To offer the opportunity to provide the right resource at the right time in right manner and
- To create a better match with the expressed needs of the users.

An assessment of the user perceptions on resources, services and needs in the sector was conducted to garner insights in improving the services and resources key to their needs. The details are given in the following sections.

Perceptions on Information Need

Perceptions of fish farmers and fishers on necessity of information in their livelihood activities were surveyed and the test result is summarized in figure 15 below. It was surveyed whether they need information for their livelihood activities on the ratings (1) very essential (2) essential (3) important (4) necessary and (5) not necessary. Seventy four fish farmers and twenty six fishers took part in the survey consider information is very essential for their livelihood activities and in making profit. However a small number of fishers consider information from an external source not necessary in their farming/ fishing activities and profit making. In general, fish farmers perceive information very essential for success of various processes of their entrepreneurial activities.

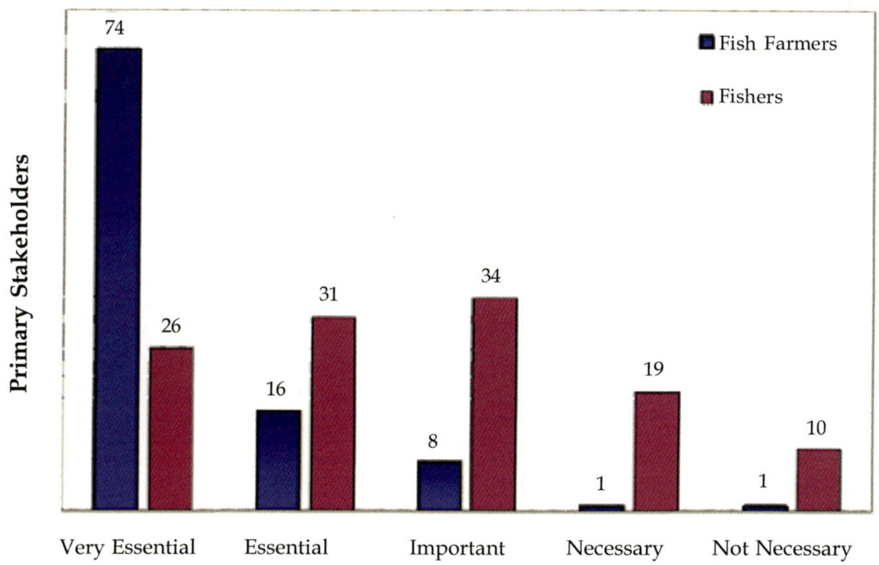

Figure 15. Perceptions of primary stakeholders on Need of Information

In fish farming sector, major demand for information caters to small-scale group (56 %) and only 8% constitute information for large scale fish farming (Figure 16).

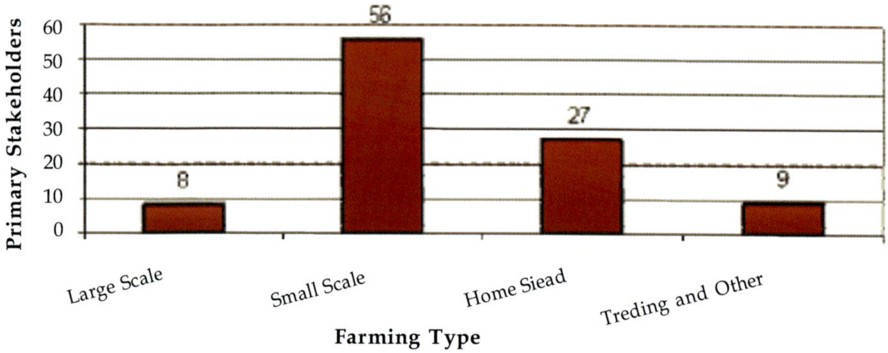

Figure 16. Information Needs on various Fish Farming groups

Information on small scale followed by homestead fish farming was in need by the farmers. Information needs of fish farmers regarding fish species selection, fish breeding, fish disease and disaster management, farm implements, sustainable fish farming etc were collected and summarized in Figure 17. Summary figure shows that the information requirements of fishers and fish farmers are differing. This is due to differences in their operations. Fish farming is an effort to manage a biological process but capture fishery is beyond control. Both categories of respondents are wary of marketing, weather, and information on subsidies. Fish farmers are in need of marketing, disease, species, seed, feed, disaster, scheduling of farm operations, and welfare schemes/subsidies/insurance. They needed information on all farm related activities with minor variations. Knowledge of fish physiology and biology is vital to fish farmers whereas capture fishers ignore it. However, technologies, seasons, gears, etc., are vital in fish farming as well as in fishing. The fishers and the fish farmers are equally concerned in market and other allied information once their product is harvested.

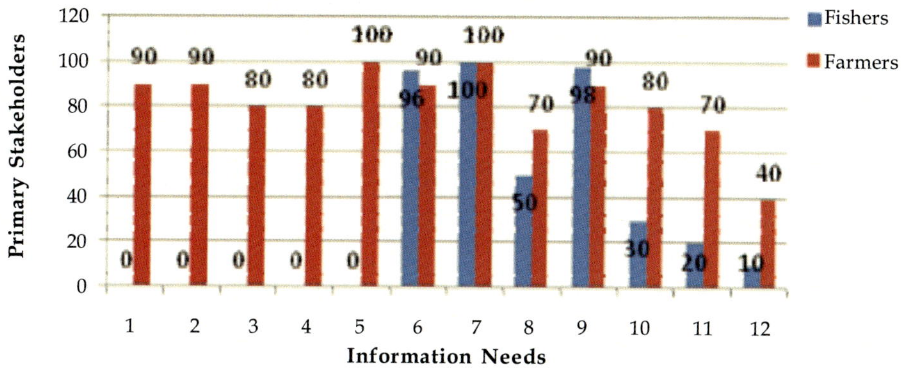

Figure 17. Information Needs on Fishing and Farm Related Activities

Legend 1. Seed/Feed Selection and Suitability; 2. Scheduling of Farm Operations; 3. Fertilizer/Feed/Medicine Application; 4. Breeding/Culture/Rearing; 5. Disease; 6. Weather/Disaster Warning; 7. Market Related; 8. Machines/Implements; 9. Schemes/ Subsidies/Insurance; 10. Responsible farming/fishing; 11. Ancillary/Allied Operations; 12. Other

Fish farming (aquaculture) and fishing differs in many aspects. If fishing can be equated to hunting activity, aquaculture is agriculture involving cultivation of fish in a fixed location. Fish, like cattle or sheep, have to be fed and cared for. Like the crop producer, the fish farmer has to be concerned with the growth and timing of the harvest. Fishing entails only harvesting, the rest taken care of by nature itself. The overall findings clearly highlight the deficiencies in information services rendered by agencies concerned in the sector. As a whole, need-based and demand-driven information services are deficient in the sector, especially on small scale and homestead farming.

Perception on Information Sources

The primary stakeholders were surveyed to know their perceptions on the media as sources they rely on for fishery information and the results are summarized in the figure 18 below. For farmers, Internet, personal ways and libraries are the sources of information in that sequence. Majority of the fishers rely on mobile phones, followed by personal ways and other means for gathering information. Use of Internet sources was higher among fish farmers in comparison with the fishers. This indicates the need for ICT based certified contents services for the benefit of fish farmers. It is also noted that certain population of primary stakeholders do not know source media like information kiosk, Village Knowledge Centre, fish clinic *etc.* in the sector.

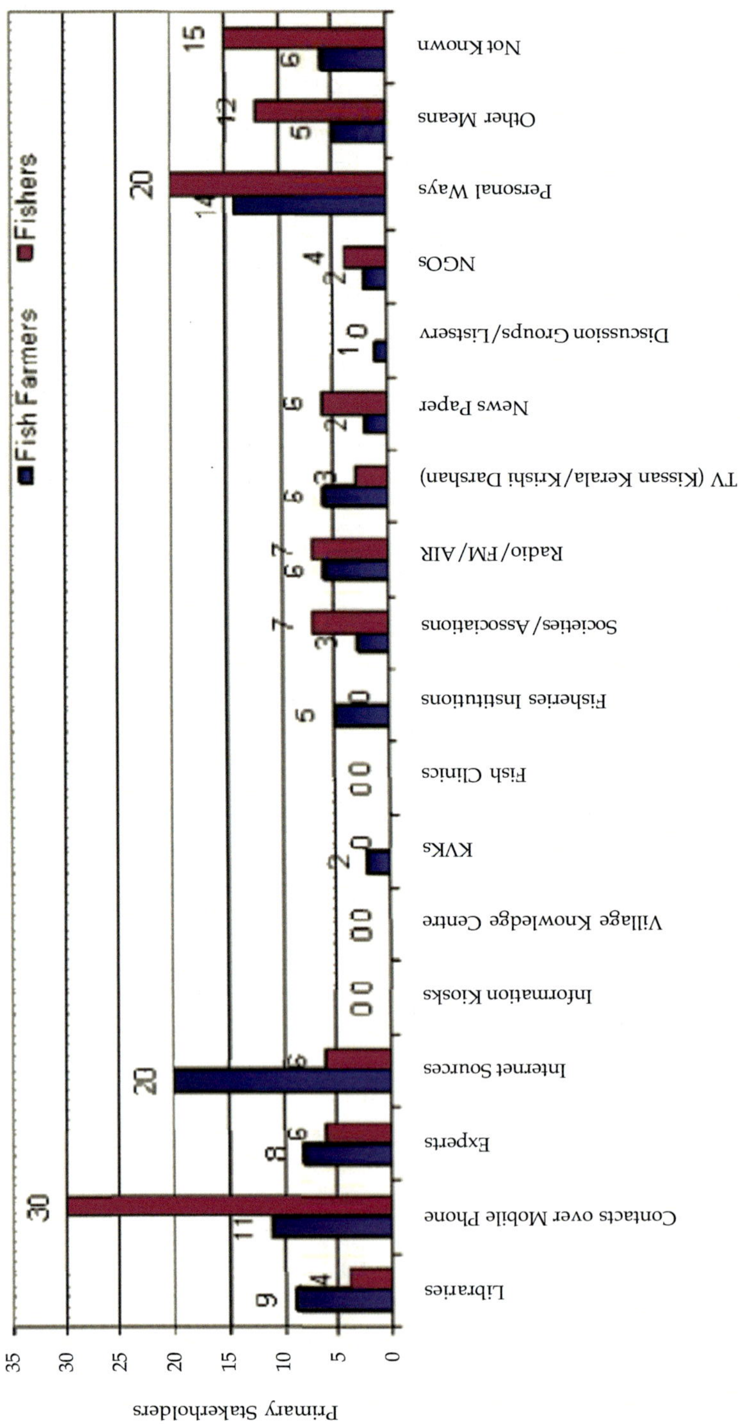

Figure 18. Information Sources Preferred by Primary Stakeholders

Perception on Information Services

The perceptions of the fish farmers and fishers with respect to the effectiveness and usefulness of information systems and services in the sector in general was surveyed and the result is presented in figure 19 below. The test was conducted on the ratings (1) very good (2) good (3) satisfactory (4) inferior (5) bad and (6) no rating. Majority of the respondents rated the information systems and services as satisfactory and inferior. Majority of fishers could not give rating on the systems and services as its existence were not known to them. The test results indicate the need for introduction of new services and a system for barrier free flow of information, oriented towards the requirements of the primary stakeholders in the sector.

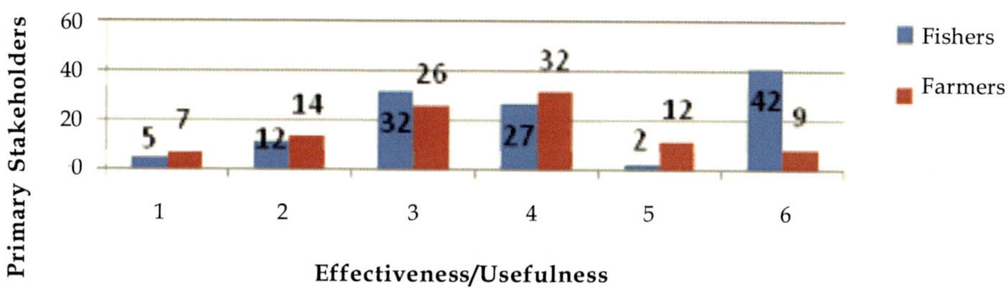

Figure 19. Usefulness of Information Services

Legend : 1: Very Good; 2: Good; 3: Satisfactory; 4: Inferior; 5: bad; 6:No Rating

Preferences of the primary stakeholders on access to information resources and services were surveyed and the results are depicted in figure 20 below. The test included access points that are related to their livelihood activities such as (1) fisheries institution libraries (2) village libraries/VKCs/societies/*Akshaya centres;* (3) *Matsya Bhavans*/Board/Department offices and (4) NGOs. The results show that the fishers prefer to the grassroot level institution viz NGOs, village libraries, societies, etc. over the government offices and institutional libraries. NGOs have scored excellent rating followed by village libraries/VKCs/socities. Majority of them rated the Matsya Bhavans/ Board/Dept. offices as poor and inferior in relying for information.

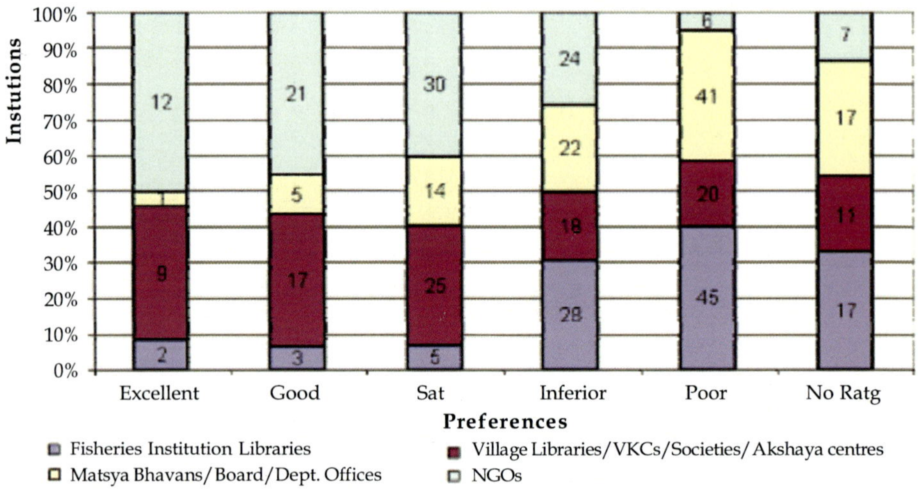

Figure 20. Preferences of Fish Farmers for Information Access

The same test was conducted separately for fish farmers as the information requirements in the farming operations differ from fishing operations and the test results are summarized in the figure 21 below.

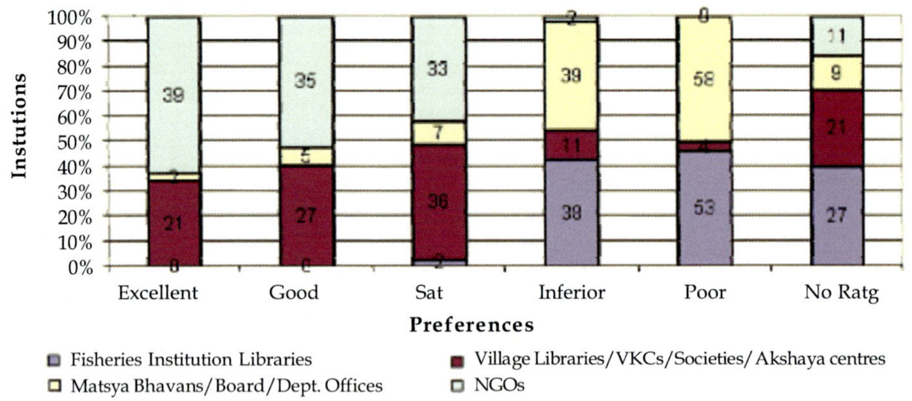

Figure 21. Preferences of Fishers on Institutional Facilities for Information Access

The test results reveal that village level information centres and NGO centres are preferred by fishers over institutional libraries and government department offices. The tests indicate that the grass-root level institutions like NGOs, village libraries, primary societies, etc. are preferred by the primary stakeholders over the government offices and institional libraries as an information resource centre. It also points to the need of revamping information services meant for primary stakeholders in the government offices, institutions and libraries.

Deficiency in Information Services in the Sector

Expected or anticipated services needed by the primary stakeholders differ from that of scientists, teachers, researchers and students. Evaluation was done using Mann-Whiteney test to know whether there was any significant difference between two group viz. fish farmers and fishers with regard to their needs for information services deficient thereto. The service criteria were (1) training on new technological information (2) weather warning in mass media/ mobile; (3) simple printed materials in local language on scientific matters (4) single window information gateways on fishery related matters (5) accessibility to Help Desk, experts and other sources of information and (6) accessibility to market / farming/ fishery/ finance/ welfare related information on Internet/ Mobile in local language. The rating criteria for the test were (1) highly needed (2) much needed (3) needed (4) low need (5) not needed and (6) no rating. The box plot of the test is given as Figure 22.

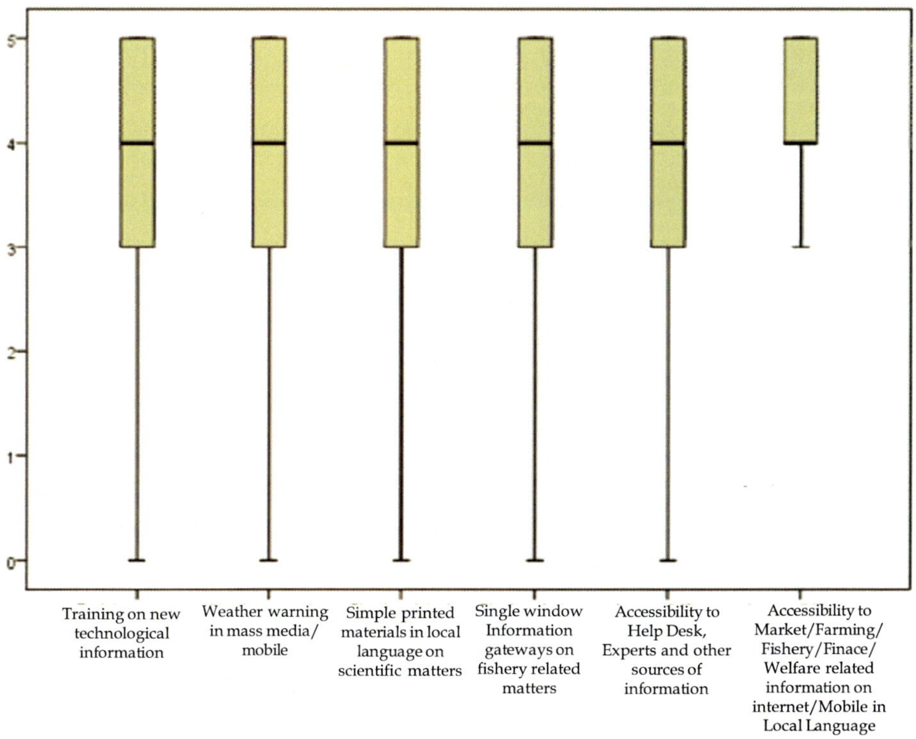

Figure 22. Information Service Needs

All the categories have median value of 4. Need for market/ farming/fishery/finance/welfare related information on Internet/ mobile in local language is rated precisely by the stakeholders.

Awareness of Advisory Services

Awareness of the fish farmers and fishers on various information/ advisory services operational in the sector were evaluated. The result is presented in figure 23. Welfare, weather (Ocean State Forecast (OSF)) and Preferred Fishing Zone (PFZ) service of INCOIS are known to 30-40% of fishers surveyed. Welfare and weather information are known to 25-30% of fish farmers surveyed. However, awareness of fisheries and marketing related information are low among both fish farmers and fishers. OSF and PFZ are highly innovative, ICT driven and are disseminated over a wide spectrum of media and therefore, awareness of these services is high among the stakeholders. It is evident that integration and harmonization of media, technology and information contents give birth to effective information services and the sector is in need of similar types of services especially in fisheries information, marketing information and agro advisory information services.

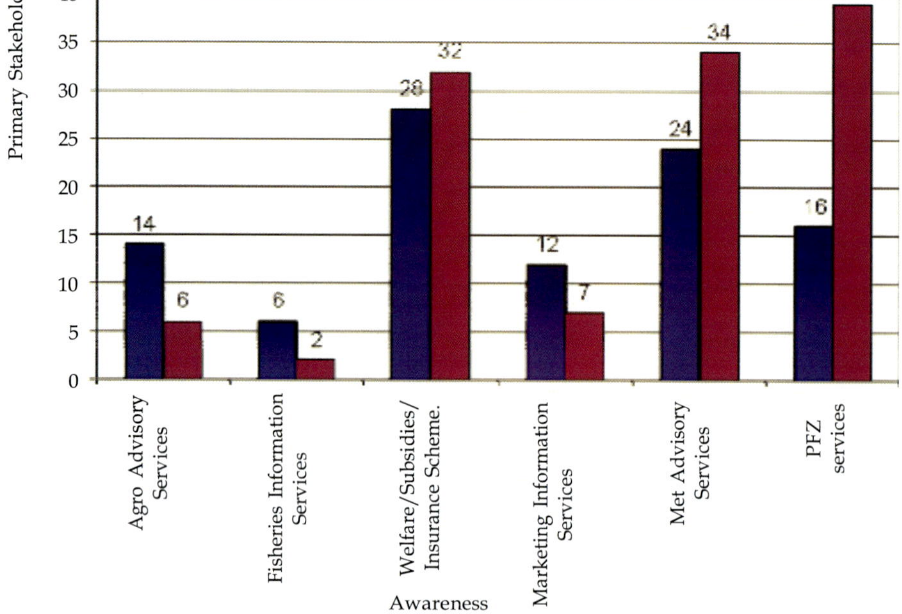

Figure 23. Awareness o f Advisory Services

Media Preferred

Perceptions on the media preferrd by the primary stakeholders for receiving information were surveyed and the results are summarized in figure 24 below. Among the primary stakeholders, fishers preferred mobile phones (50%) and fish farmers preferred Internet based services (30%). Television and radio are also popular among them. Media remain important for access and utilization of information services. Introduction of mobile based services such as Simple Message Services (SMS), alerts on inclement weather conditions, cash transactions from societies or government welfare funds into the bank account of the farmer, etc. can help them saving time and efforts. Such services can also sensitize them on newer media of information services in the offing.

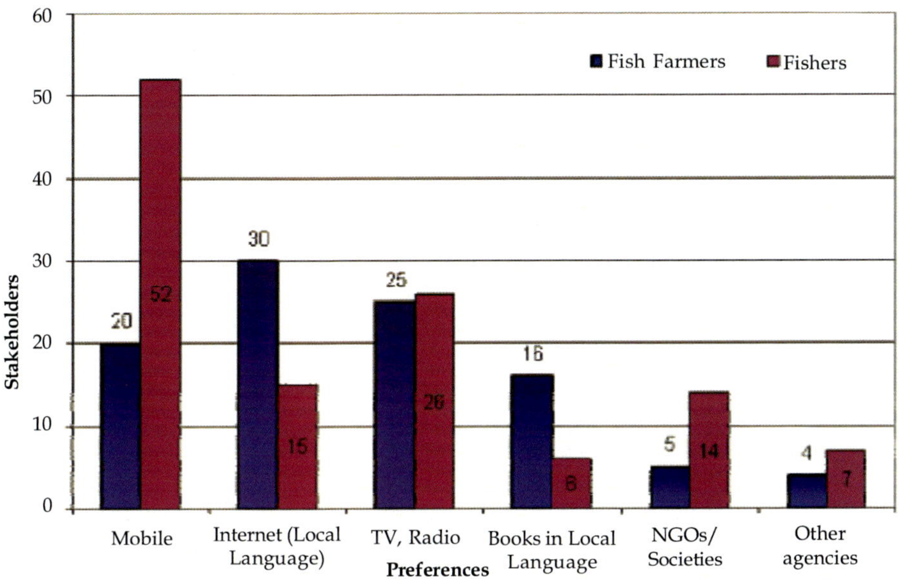

Figure 24. Media Preferred by Farming and Fishing Communities

State government can collaborate with and seek expertise of NGOs in setting up Village Knowledge Centres (VKCs). The best model in this regard is MS Swaminathan Research Foundation (MSSRF) which provides information services to the fishing community in selected regions. The Department-NGO relations should be promoted in designing and implementing information dissemination services instead of the bureaucratic ridden, no-demand driven; no-diffusion media based; non-absorbent content driven; non-comprehensible language driven information services.

Critical Assessment on Fisheries Information Sources and Services

Test for critical assessment on information sources and services offered to the primary stakeholders were carried out on the indicators of (1) no spreading of awareness (2) diverse sources (3) institutional sources non reachable (4) local language disregarded in ICT based services and (5) information services are not user driven and not demand driven. Test results are presented in Figure 25. The analysis shows that information provisions to both categories of primary stakeholders viz., fishers and fish farmers are vulnerable. The vehement expressions are above 50% on all the criteria put to test. Disregard of local language in ICT based services scored the highest voted by fish farmers and fishers. Diverse sources, non reachable institutions, lack of awareness on sources, scant regard to the primary stakeholders in the design of information services, etc. are other problems in the sector.

The results suggest for effective, efficient and content based fisheries information services designed for the primary stakeholders also. Digital and other electronic technologies are transforming our economies, societies and ways of living. Technology has had an especially profound impact on the information and communication activities that have always been central to sustainable development. Agricultural Information Services in vague do not amply cover fisheries sector.

Library and information systems can play crucial roles for delivery of services because libraries are the important tool or agencies for information delivery and for guiding users through the maze of complex sources of information. Appropriate communication and networking methods enable better reach of knowledge and information to the target audiences including improved access to print and electronic material in local languages. *Kissan Kerala,* the ICT enabled service operational in farming sector offers new dimensions in providing information services.

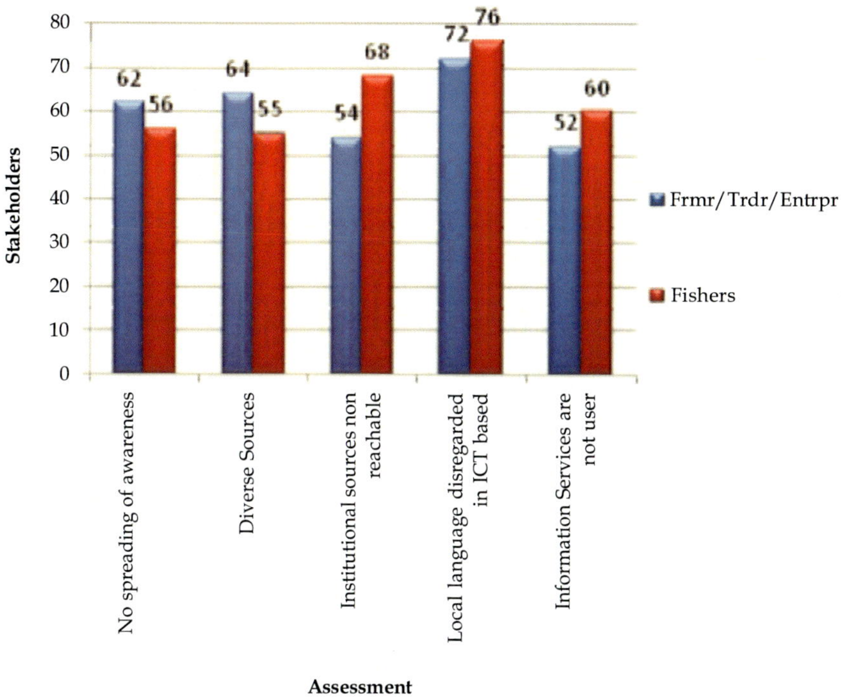

Figure 25. Critical Assessment on Information Sources and Services

The overall situation in the Department of Fisheries, Government of Kerala suggests that the department does not acknowledge the library and information system as an agency of transformation in the sector. Fisheries information distribution in Kerala State is weak, moribund and conventional. The dynamic information provision is absent even in the Home pages of the Department of Fisheries of Kerala State. Nevertheless, the Web page of the Fisheries Department put bombastic words reading -*'with the complexity in technology the task of dissemination of knowledge and skill become complex which warrants sustained and systematic efforts on the part of Department of Fisheries'* (NIFAM 2013). Information on fisheries schemes and programmes are inaccessible over modern communication media and they reside in the registers and files of *Matsya Bhavans*, FFDA etc. In fact the Kerala State Fisheries Department which has to serve the user community ten times more in quantity than other institutions has inadequate information resources and services. The Department needs Cyber systems and implementation of information exchange programmes for optimal utilization of information resources. As

Mobile phones are the powerful hand held computing machines which can provide means for faster communication of information on fisheries practices, ocean warning, weather information, market prices, water specific and region specific fisheries information, services based on mobile telephony are also to be implemented in the sector. Measures to meet the information needs of small-scale fishing communities and fish farmers are inadequate and critical in the state. The state of affairs discussed above cannot be different in other States of India also.

Enterprises in fisheries sector such as fishing and fish farming (aquaculture) would be seen not only as a technical and biological innovation, but also as a socio-economic enterprise that requires the same kind of social analyses, services and systems as any other production system. The policy makers should prompt to introduce information services providing single window access to information in a cohesive manner. The dynamic trends and advancements in ICT make it possible for such services. To materialize, larger participation of LIS professionals as in any information system is needed. Equal opportunity to access information is important for the fishing community also as for the research or business patron in fisheries sector. As technology is ready, an information system dedicated to the fisheries sector, not only in Kerala, but also whole India, ensuring equitable access to fisheries information needs implementation.

The State of Kerala do not have an institute envisioned as a Centre of Excellence in Tropical Fishery to provide scientific support for government decision making on matters related to fishery, with particular emphasis on conservation, sustainable utilization, scientific management of fishery resources, fishery economics, socio-techno-politico and cultural impacts in fisheries sector, etc. Sri C Achutha Menon, the visionary Chief Minister of Kerala was instrumental in starting number of institutions such as KFRI, CDS, CESS, CWRDM, KAU, Sri Chithirathirunal Centre for Medical Science, Kerala Electronic Development Corporation (Keltron), etc. These institutions also advice the Government on specific issues related to their subjects. Scientific advices rendered by a university or an expert may need further examination on its implications as well. On the matters of fisheries, the State government is advised by Advisor to the Government and institutions such as CDS for decision making. The State does not have a Centre of Excellence on Fisheries to give scientific support for government decision making. Therefore, the State of Kerala may institute Kerala Fisheries Informatics and Research Institute as

Centre of Excellence to provide scientific information support to the government on issues related to fisheries and to address problems in the fisheries information cycle, dissemination, access, consolidation and services, notwithstanding KUFOS and other Central Institutions in Kerala.

❑❑❑

Chapter-7

Qualitative Evaluation of Fisheries Information Capacity

Patrons' views are very important in studies related to information systems and services. The information stakeholders have their own distinct and different perspectives on library and information resources, services and systems. Quantitative evaluations carried out in previous sections have further been evaluated qualitatively in order to get realistic view of the matter under investigation so that possible solutions could be suggested for the problems and inefficiencies if any found in the system. The user categories overlap many times as a scientist may be a teacher and an extension worker also. Care is taken, as far as possible to count a user in the most general category in the case of multi roles. In student category, PG students and in researcher category, PhD Scholars are considered for the survey. The term 'capacity' refers to the ability or power to contain, absorb or hold maximum volume or amount of information resources and infrastructure. As the libraries are the agencies for delivery of information to the users, 'information capacity' refers to the resources and services that are measured through library and information systems operating in the sector. Qualitative data was collected from 14 top officials of the National and the State fisheries institutions on various aspects of library and information systems with the objective of validating findings dealt in the previous Chapters. Users groups of fisheries information consist of the following:

1. Students
2. Scientists
3. Officers
4. Researchers
5. Teachers

6. Extension workers
7. Fish farmers
8. Fishers
9. Entrepreneurs and
10. People's representatives

Information Sources

The study identified indicators of fisheries information sources for the stakeholders as:

1. Personal Contacts
2. Library Resources
3. Institutional Resources
4. Web Resources
5. Government Resources and
6. Other

User views on above indicators were obtained and test was conducted by applying Kruskal-Wallis test. The box plot Figure 26 shows that library resources, personal contacts and institutional resources had median of 3, government resources 2, and Web resources 4. Though library resources are the preferred source by the students, teachers, scientists and researchers, median value of 4 to web resources indicates importance of web based information services in the sector. Analysis of the test revealed that the library resources are the preferred source of information by all user groups except fishers and farmers. Officers opted for government resources; students, researchers, scientists and teachers preferred library resources. Personal contacts and web resources formed the preferred source of information by the fishers, fish farmers, NGO workers and people's representatives. It indicates the need of strengthening different resources as well as integration of all categories of resources for effective use and availability of information to all types of user groups.

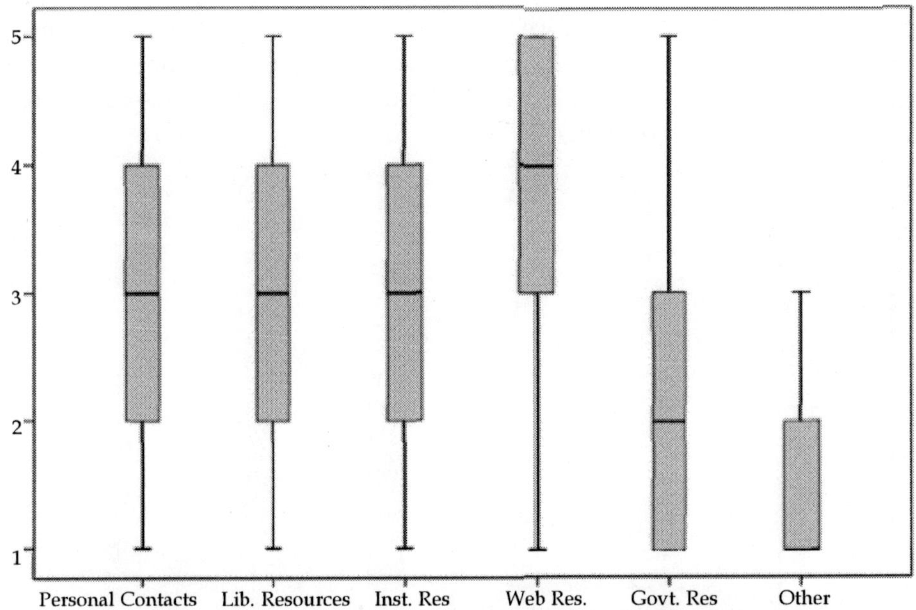

Figure 26. Test of Significance of Information Sources

Library Resources

The main information resource indicators of fisheries sector identified by the study are:

1. Books
2. Periodicals
3. Back Volumes (BVs)
4. Electronic Information Sources (EIS)
5. Web
6. Fisheries Data

The opinion of users on the above indicators in terms of their preferences to those resources was obtained and put to test by using Kruskal-Wallis test. It is evident that books and periodicals are the preferred sources by the scientists, teachers, students and researchers. However, fishers and fish farmers are not concerned with the periodicals, bound volumes of journals, EIS, and fisheries data. The box plot Figure 27 shows median 3 on books and periodicals and median 2 with rest of the groups. Uneven quartile groups show very different distributions of views. Tall box plot for periodical and Web suggests that it is source of information but the median value of these two suggests a difference between groups. It is revealed that resources in all diversity are used by the stakeholders, every resource its reader and every reader its resource.

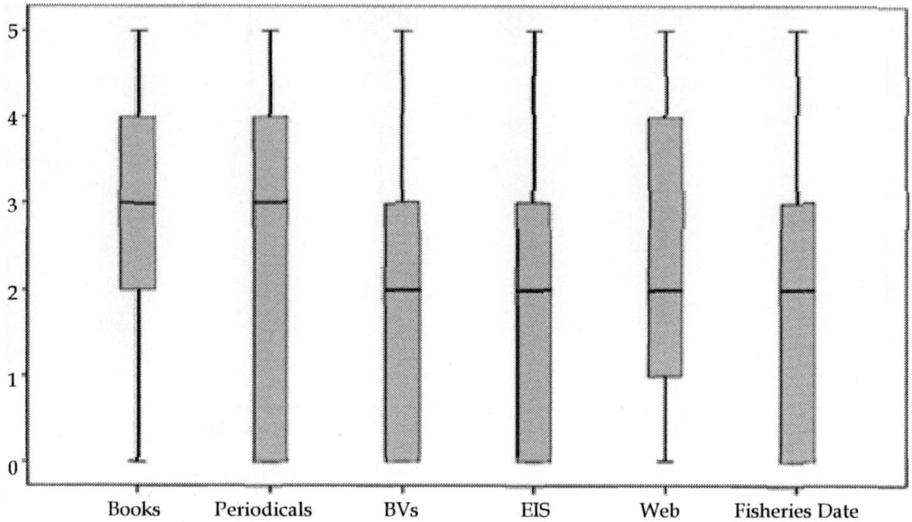

Figure 27. Test of Significance of Library Resources

Information Services

The information services indicators identified by the study are:

1. Reference Services
2. Information Services
3. OPAC
4. Current Awareness Service (CA)
5. Selective Dissemination of Information (SDI) and
6. Orientation on Information Services

User views on the above indicators in terms of the significance they attach to those services was obtained and put to test by using Kruskal-Wallis test. The users consisting of scientists, teachers, students and researchers opined OPAC service, reference services and information services rendered by library and information sector as Good. The box plot Figure 28 shows that the OPAC has median of 4 with upper quartile 5 and lower quartile 3. Reference, Information and OPAC has median 4, SDI has median 3 with lower quartile 0,

Current Awareness Service and orientation with median 3. The analysis indicates that Orientation, SDI and Current Awareness services have to be given due importance by the libraries in introducing information services and resources to the user groups from time to time. It also shows that SDI services are not generally provided in the fisheries libraries. Similarly, Reference, Information and OPAC services have to be further strengthened in the sectoral libraries.

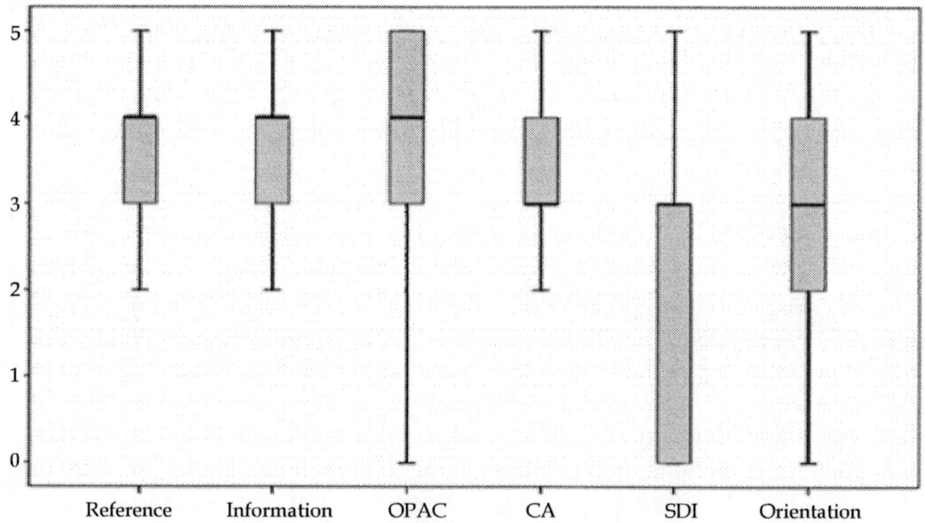

Figure 28. Test of Significance of Information Services

IT Enabled Information Services

IT enabled information services have become very important in the libraries. The study identified indicators of IT enabled services as follows:

1. CDROM Database Search Services
2. Online Database Search Services
3. Digital Repository Services
4. e-Book services and
5. e-Journal services

The opinion of sectoral users on the above indicators in terms of the significance they attach to those services was obtained and put to test by using Kruskal-Wallis test. The box plot Figure 29 shows that user views are varied on the significance of IT enabled information services rendered in the sector. The most accessed EIS are e-Journals. There are significant difference with respect to E-books, Digital Repositories and Online Databases. CDROM search, Online database search and Digital Repositories in the sector show the medium of 3. Box plot shows that there is a wide range of preferences for online database search and E-books have a low profile in the sector.

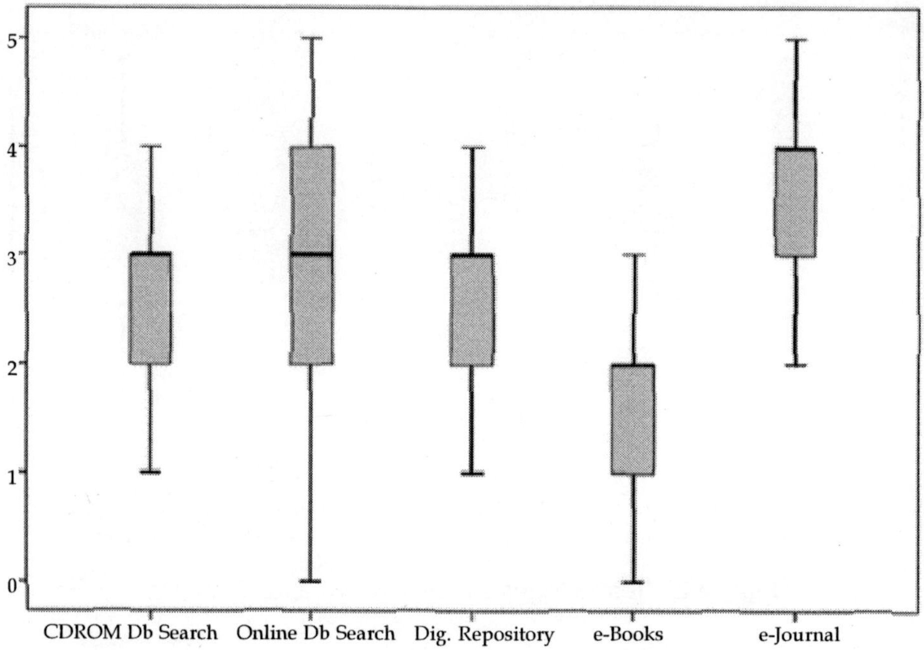

Figure 29. Test of Significance of IT Enabled Information Services

Library System Components

The library system components indicators are:

1. Staff competency
2. Different abilities of the professionals such as communication
3. Routine services rendered by the library
4. Maintenance and upkeep of the library
5. Information services and tools offered in the library
6. Ambience and physical facilities of the library and
7. Orientation/training offered by the library.

These indicators were tested on the user categories viz., (1) scientists (2) teachers (3) researchers and (4) students by using Kruskal-Wallis test with the indicator ratings (1) excellent (2) very good (3) satisfactory (4) inferior (5) poor and (6) no ratings. The test revealed that the staff, services, maintenance and ambience in the library and information divisions are good but information services and orientation offered are significantly different below 0.05. Box plot Figure 30 shows that all the components have a high level of agreement except orientation/training imparted in fisheries libraries.

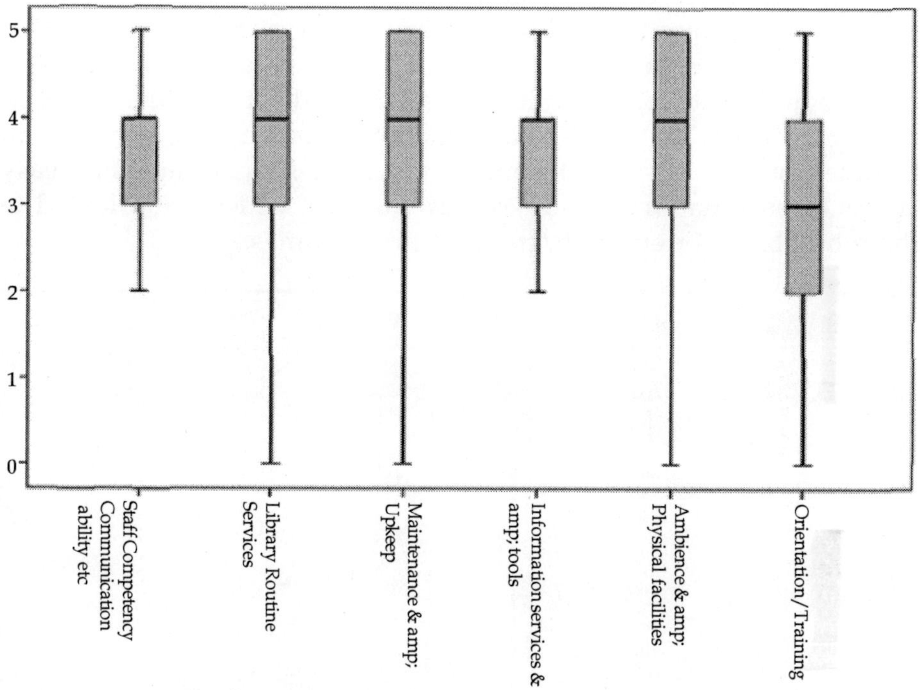

Figure 30. Test of Significance of LIS Components

Access to Resources and Services

The study identified the following indicators for measuring the capacity of the sector for access to information resources and services:

1. Orientation on fisheries information sources, systems and services
2. Acquisition of new resources especially on Fish Health, deep sea resources, bio-energetics and marine phycology
3. Innovative ICT based information dissemination services

4. Digitization of TK, Grey literature, and institutional wisdom
5. User authenticated access to e-resources
6. Access to documents of other institutions/resource sharing/inter library loan

These indicators were tested with the user categories viz., (1) scientists (2) teachers (3) researchers and (4) students by using Kruskal-Wallis test. For the test, the ratings scales (1) excellent (2) very good (3) satisfactory (4) inferior (5) poor and (6) no ratings are used. The box plot (Figure 31) reveals that that there is a high level of agreement with the user groups regarding the capacity for access to information resources and services in the sector with median value of 4 and lower quartile at 3 with regard to almost all the indicators. There is need among the users for access to information resources of institutions in fisheries and allied sector through innovative services enabling easy access to information, resources, new subjects which are oriented to them by library orientation/training programmes.

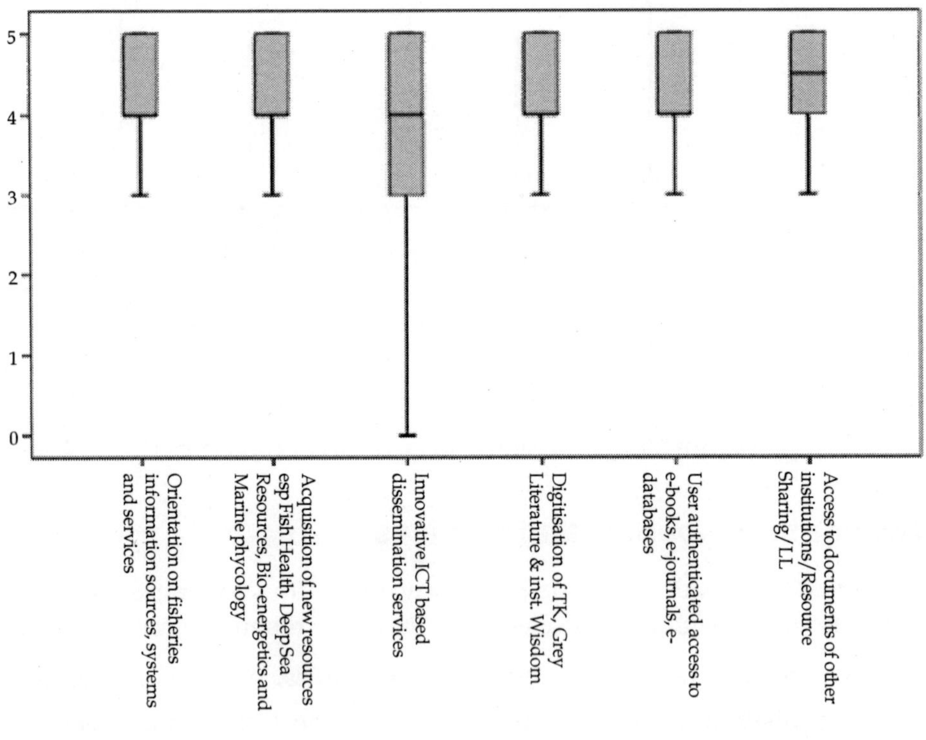

Figure 31. Test of Significance of Access to Resources and Services

International, Regional and National Fisheries Information Services

Opinion on the access and use of the international, regional and national fisheries information services on Web as indicated below were tested by using Kruskal-Wallis test:

1. FAO and sub-sets
2. WFC, WAS, ICSF
3. NACA, PIMRIS
4. Government of India Portal
5. Agrisnet/Agmarknet
6. Agropedia
7. CeRA
8. ICAR
9. National Fisheries Institutions
10. eprints@cmfri
11. INCOIS
12. NARS, IMD

The results on information service categories listed in Figure 32 indicate very different distributions of views of the user group viz., (1) scientists (2) teachers (3) researchers (4) students and (5) officers. FAO and its sub sets, CeRA, National Fisheries Institutions and Government of India Portal have a range of users but have median value of 3 and 2 only. *Agropedia* and web services of ICAR have median 1 and other national and regional services have median 2. The low median value indicates low utilization of services by the user categories. It is also revealed that scientists and teachers give higher ratings for FAO and CeRA, officers give higher rating to Government of India Portal, students and researchers give higher ratings to CeRA and E-Prints@CMFRI.

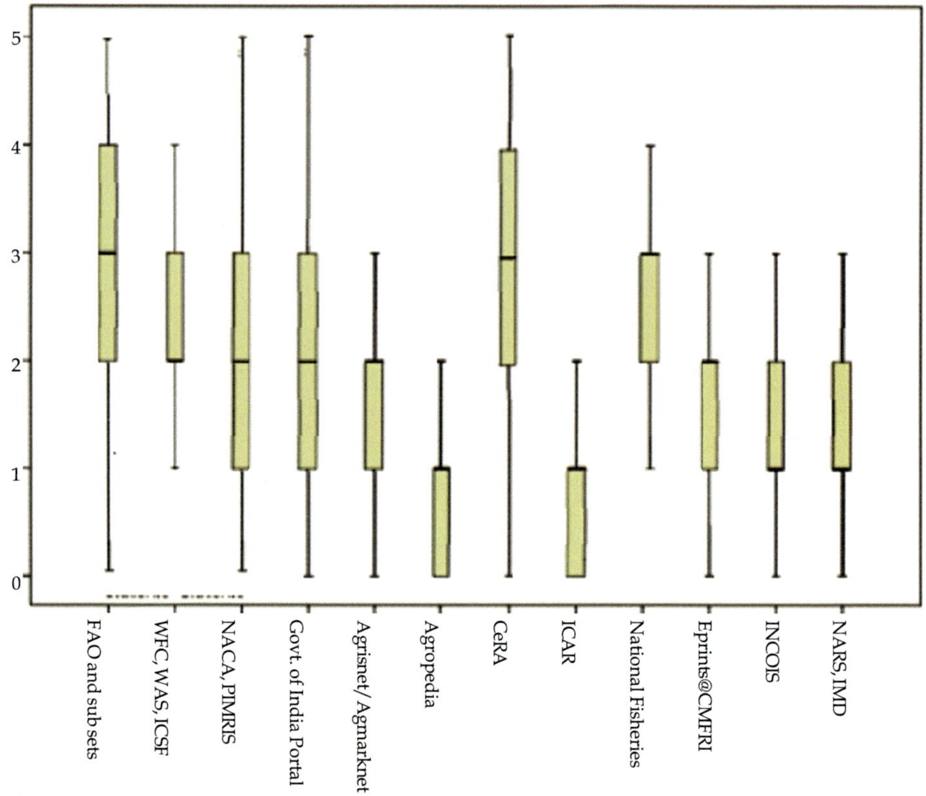

Figure 32. Test of Significance of Access and Use of International, Regional and National Information Services

Qualitative Evaluation

Indicators were formulated and included in the Questionnaire/ Interview Schedule prepared for Top level officers of the sector and the results could be measured to crosscheck and corroborate the facts found in the earlier tests. Following sections give details of the tests conducted.

Fisheries Information Sub Sectors

The study identified following seven indicators of fisheries information sub-sectors and a test was conducted to evaluate the strength and weakness of these sub-sectors by seeking opinion of the top officers in the sector:

1. Bibliographic
2. Management

3. Extension
4. Scientific
5. Statistical
6. Decision support and
7. Experts in the sector

Evaluating the strength of fisheries information sub-sectors shall be helpful in managing and developing them in a sustainable way. The results of the test are summarized in Figure 33. Bibliographic information and Experts as source of information are strong in the sector (77 percent). Scientific Information sector is the only indicator which got Very Strong rating though constitute 8 percentage (n=13). In an overall analysis, the information sub-sectors such as scientific, bibliographic and experts are satisfactory in the sector in terms of their information capacity. Extension, Statistical and Decision Support information sub-sectors are weak in the sector and need strengthening.

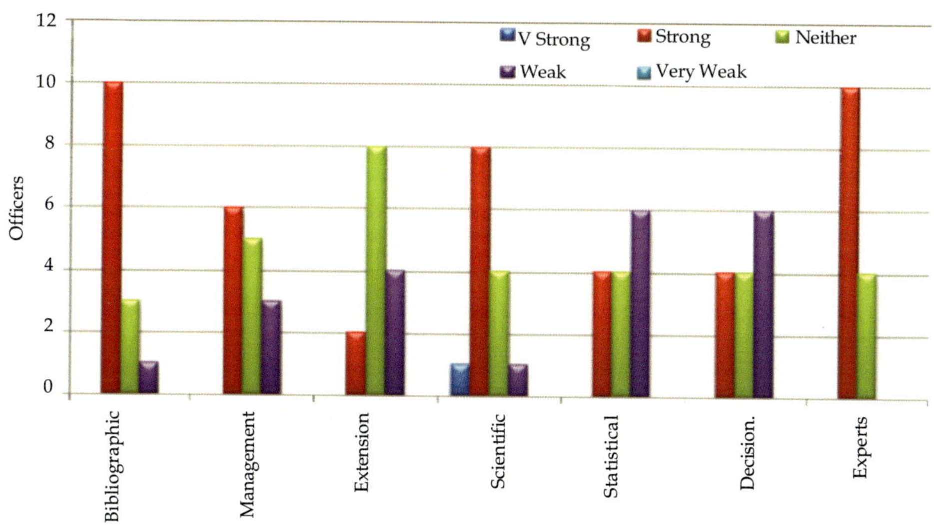

Figure 33. Information Capacity of Fisheries Sub-Sectors

Fisheries Information Domains

Evaluating the strength of information domains shall be helpful in managing and developing them in a sustainable way. The study identified following eight indicators as Fisheries information domains:

1. Fishery and Operations

2. Fishery Biology and Environment
3. Economics and Finance
4. Socio-Economic
5. Socio-Cultural
6. Legal
7. Fish Health
8. Aqua Farming

A test was conducted by seeking opinion of the officers at the helm of affairs to evaluate the strength of these domains in terms of information capacity. The test is summarized in Figure 34. Bibliographic information and Experts as source of information are strong in the sector (77 percent). Scientific Information sector is the only indicator which got Very Strong rating though constitute 8 percentage (n=13). Fishery and Operations (F & Op). Fishery Biology and Environment (Bio & Env) are the two domains with 31 percentage of Very Strong and 77 percentage of Strong ratings. Economics and Finance (Econ & Fin) information domain is also strong in the sector. Legal, Socio-Economic (Soc-Econ) and Socio-Cultural (Soc-Cul) information domains are weak. Fish Health and Aqua Farming Information domains are very weak. Very weak information capacity indicates the criticality in the management of fish diseases, farming operations, socio-economic-cultural schemes in the sector.

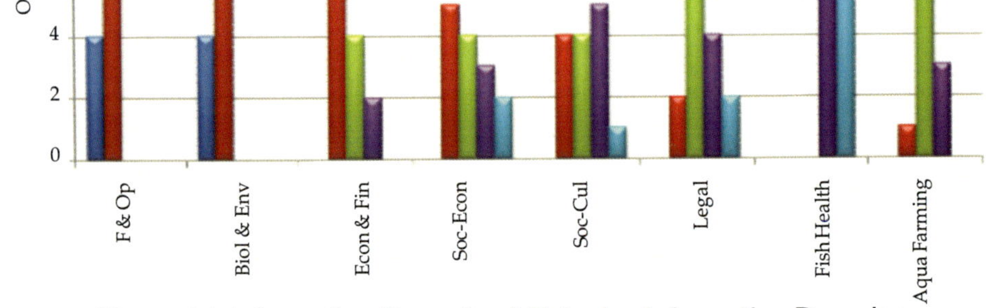

Figure 34. Information Capacity of Fisheries Information Domains

Critical Gaps and Deficiencies

The indicators formulated by the study on critical gaps in information infrastructure of fisheries sector are:

1. Lack of reliable data
2. Weak multi-disciplinary approach
3. Weak linkage between R&D and other institutions
4. Aquaculture not treated at par with agriculture resulting into lack of resources and funds
5. Lack of sectorally targeted information
6. Weak linkages between Centre-State institutions and
7. Lack of ICT based information systems and services, GIS based inventorying of aquaculture/fisheries resources and others.

Survey was conducted to identify the critical gaps in information infrastructure indicated above. The participant officers agree with all the critical gaps in general in varying degrees. The results reveal that lack of reliable data and lack of ICT based information systems and services are the main critical gaps in the sector. As aquaculture not treated at par with agriculture, implementation of innovative information services are not given priority in the sector. Weak multi-disciplinary approach and linkages in the sector are the other two gaps prevailing in the sector. It is evident that critical gaps exist in the fisheries information domains in its various degrees and intensities. The identification of these critical gaps helps in formulating plans and programs for rectification. Evaluation is summarized in Figure 35.

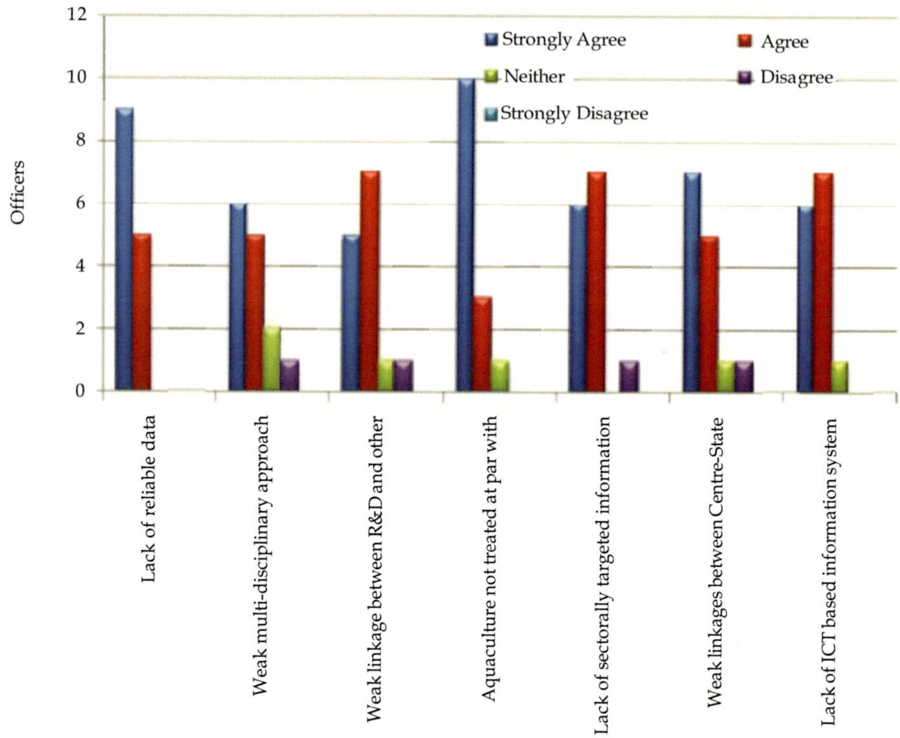

Figure 35. Critical Gaps and Deficiencies in Fisheries Information Sector

Information Dissemination

The Information sub-sectors that are operating in the fisheries sector can be grouped as follows:

1. Bibliographic
2. Management
3. Extension
4. Scientific
5. Statistical
6. Decision Support
7. Experts

A survey, seeking opinion of the officers on the capacity of these sub-sectors in terms of resources, infrastructure, information sharing and dissemination was conducted and the results are summarized in

Figure 36. The test reveals that information capacity in the sub-sector of Extension is weak, followed by the sub-sectors Statistical, Decision Support and the Experts. The Bibliographic information sub-sector shows satisfactory level of capacity. The Management, Extension and Scientific sub-sectors need further integration and strengthening. Statistical information and Decision Support Systems need planned improvement. It is evident that there is need for creating database of Experts in the specific areas, innovative dissemination mechanism in Extension, integrated statistical information services, barrier-less sharing and dissemination of data using digital technologies in all the information sub-sectors of fisheries.

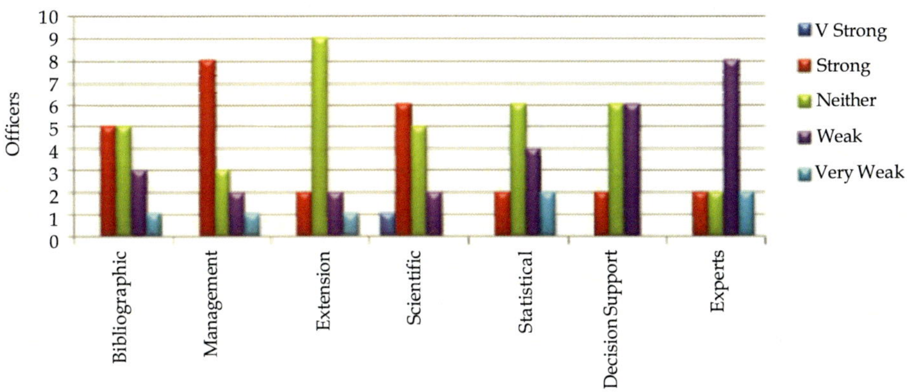

Figure 36. Information Sharing and Dissemination Capacity in Sub Sectors

Barriers

The barriers in fisheries sector for free flow of fisheries information can be listed as follows:

1. Lack of comprehensive policies
2. Compartmentalization of information
3. Incompetency in information management
4. Weightiness on tangibles rather than intangibles in information management
5. Lack of standards for information management
6. Lack of networking
7. Lack of ICT facilities and
8. Weak institutional information systems.

A survey was conducted to identify the barriers in flow of information by seeking opinion of the top officers in the sector. Though the opinions have minor variations, the test revealed that all these barriers are acting in the sector. Identification of barriers in flow of information in the sector shall help removing them. The test result is summarized in Figure 37.

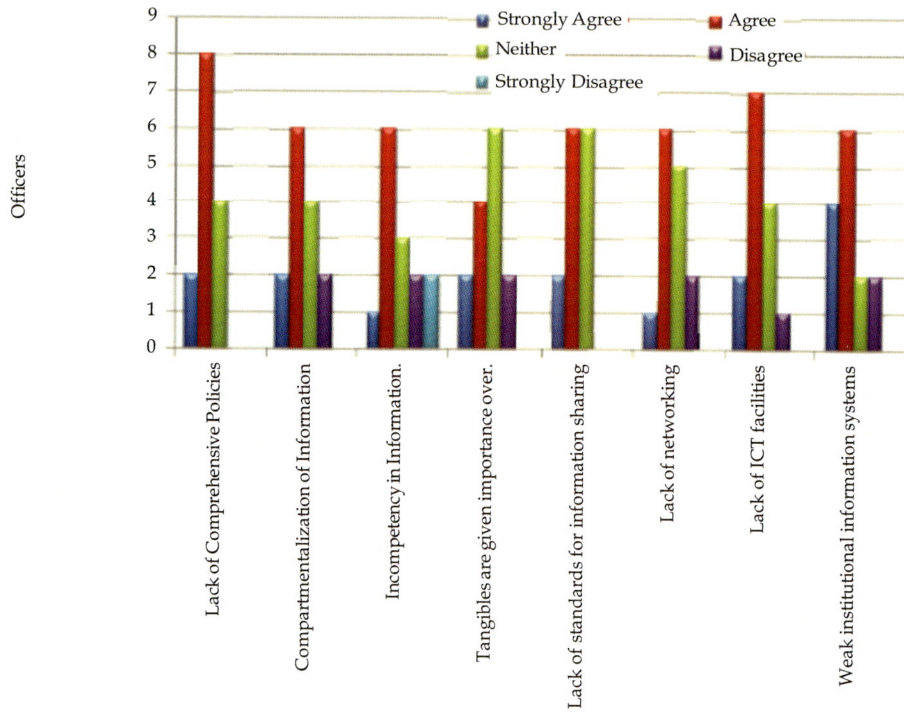

Figure 37. Barriers in Fisheries Information Sector

Information Management

The strategies for implementation of an efficient fisheries information management can be listed as follows:

1. Information capacity building
2. Utilization of the power of ICT
3. Library networking and sharing of information
4. Sectoral information systems
5. Integrated information services and
6. Delphi, Brainstorming, workshops to evolve information management programmes.

Accordingly a test was conducted in which opinions of the top officials were collected and evaluated. The results are summarized in Figure 38. It is significant to note that the opinions of the officers were almost similar in expressing the need for taking strategic measures for efficient fisheries information management especially with regard to the need of information capacity building, ICT, networking and integrated information services. The need for sectoral information systems and Delphi/Brainstorming for formulating information capacity building strategies also viewed as steps for information management in the sector. Apart from the above, the managers may have different views on the strategies for information management in the sector. The test results summarized, the factors identified in their order of priority are:

1. Integrated information services
2. Networking and sharing of information
3. Information capacity building
4. Sectoral information systems and
5. Utilization of ICT followed by
6. Need of Brain Storming, Delphi etc

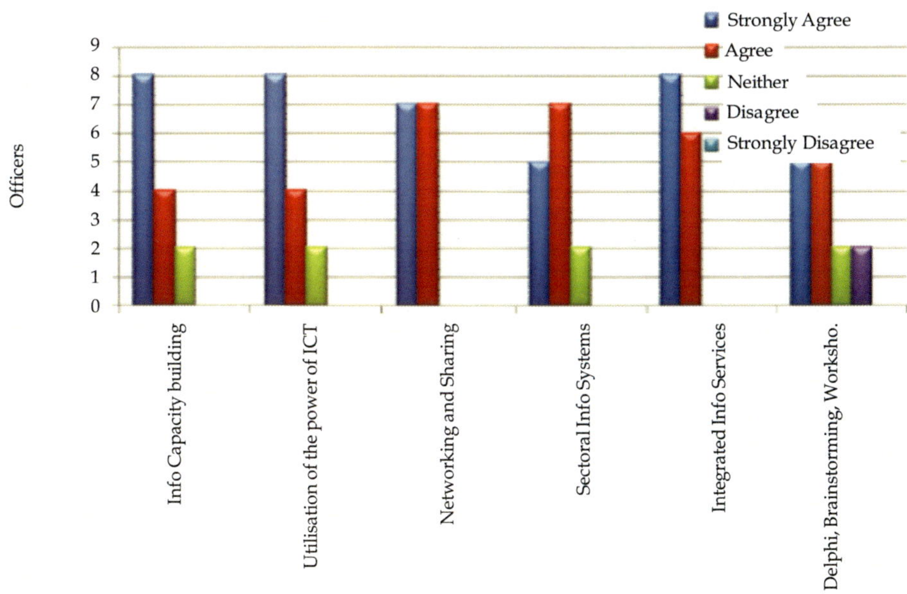

Figure 38. Strategies for Fisheries Information Management

Fisheries Information Flow

The factors that need to be fulfilled for free flow of information in the sector are:

1. Fisheries information system
2. Information network of fisheries institutions
3. An apex institution for information management
4. Centralized and closed information network of fisheries institutions and
5. De-centralized and distributed information network of fisheries institutions.

A test was conducted to garner the opinions of the top officials with respect to these factors in relation to fisheries information flow in the sector. The results indicate that the fisheries information system and fisheries information network are the steps in need, indeed for free flow of fisheries information followed by the need of an apex institution for information management. A de-centralized and distributed information network is preferred by them over a centralized and closed information network. Test result is summarized in Figure 39.

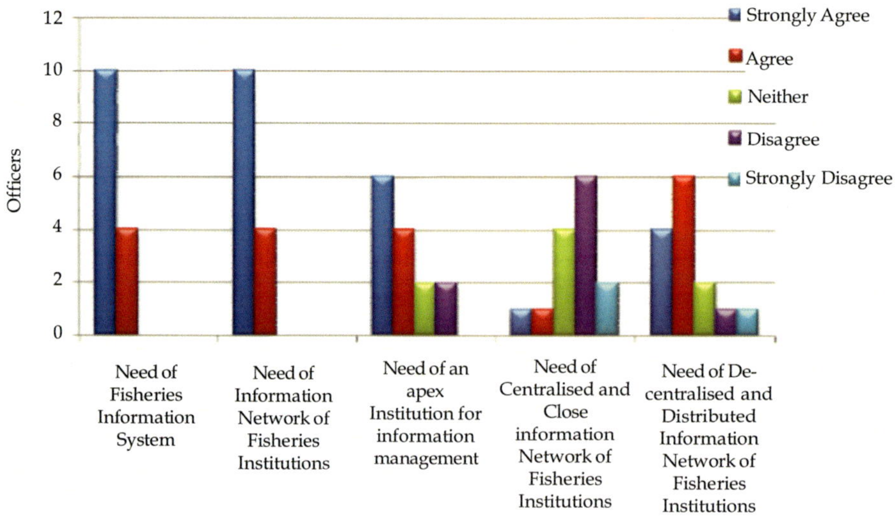

Figure 39. Steps for Free Flow of Fisheries Information

Advantages of a Dedicated Fisheries Information System

An information system is necessary for the multifarious development of fisheries sector. There shall have a profound impact on the following sectoral processes if a dedicated fisheries information system is implemented.

1. To examine processes of R&D
2. To frame holistic approach for fishery planning and development
3. To assess production potential of prospective technologies for different fishery waters and
4. To provide comprehensive and consolidated information on aforementioned aspects for all user groups.

A test was conducted seeking opinion of the top officials on the above impacts in relation to a dedicated fisheries information system and the test result is summarized in Figure 40. The results in general, indicate that activities such as research, planning, development and provisioning of information to the stakeholders shall get a fillip if a dedicated fisheries information system is put in operation in the sector.

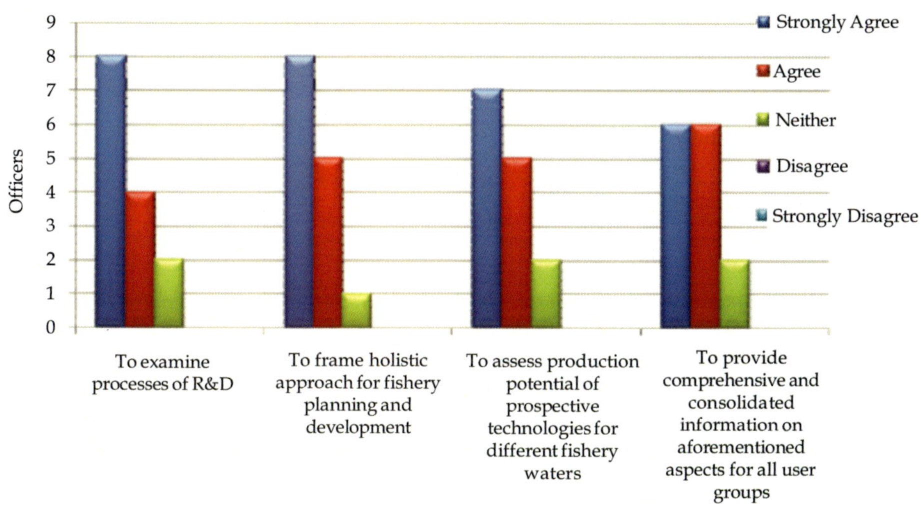

Figure 40. Advantages of a Dedicated Fisheries Information System

Knowledge Generation, Exchange and Utilization (KGEU) in Fisheries Sector

Fisheries encompass a variety of sectoral spheres. Information needs are vast and varied due to the complexity and versatility of the sector. In the sector, the Knowledge Generation, Exchange and Utilization (KGEU) processes are activated through various institutions. The basic requirement for knowledge utilization is the identification and access of appropriate information out of the multitude of resources available. Information and knowledge cannot be utilized unless they are scientifically organized. Libraries and information systems, an integral part of any knowledge management system with sophisticated tools and techniques for organization and retrieval, help in solving this problem. These systems range from simple collection of books to a computerized information system promoting transfer of information from producer to user. Information system that dictates the flow, transfer and communication of information to the user is an essential component of any knowledge dependent production.

Information Flow

Fisheries span a large resource and encompass a wide range of people. The information users in the sector comprise of the small-scale fishers making decisions about their livelihoods as well as higher officials in the ministry making plans and policies. The sources of the information are wide as shown in Figure 41.

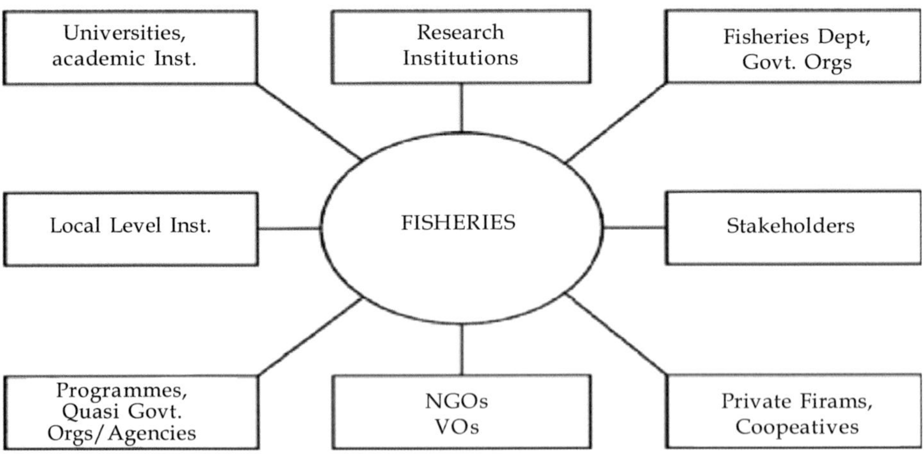

Figure 41. Information Sources in Fisheries Sector(*Source:* Sanjeeva Ghosh 2007)

Diagram showing flow of information in the sector is given in Figure 42. The flow of information is almost linear in the sector till it approaches the resource users. The dotted lines indicate a less frequent and less effective flow of fisheries information. One of the major limitations of the linear method of communication is that it denies interaction between the communicator and the receiver.

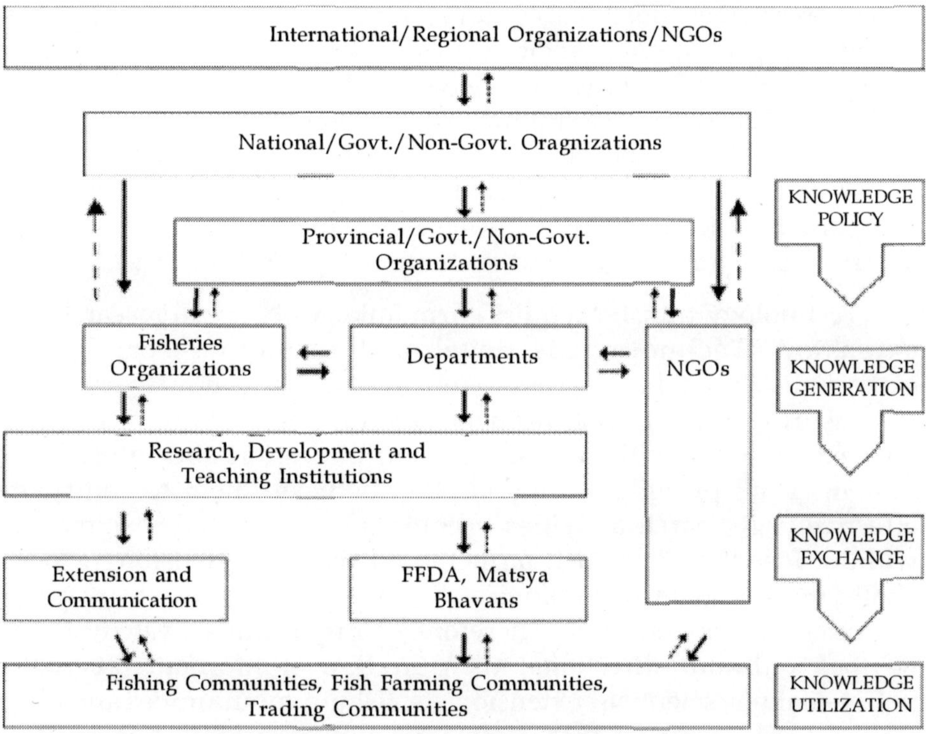

Figure 42. Flow of Information in Fisheries Sector

Dynamic Model for Knowledge Utilization

Information exchange through some system of messaging is the central theme of communication. Fisheries sector in general have a very poor and unorganized data system. Communication of data is even more critical in the sector. In order to deliver the messages effectively, the container for the message, the best channel for delivering the message, etc. are important (McConney and Haynes 2011). Appropriate communication and networking methods including improved access to print and electronic material in local languages enable better reach to target audiences. Radio, television, interactive platforms, dedicated training workshops, etc are the popular methods used in the sector. Nevertheless, the present systems are conventional and moribund in their operations and deliverance of services.

Fisheries extension tools and their multi-dimensional applications are important in the management and conservation of Open Access fishery resources, sustainable development, conflict resolution and maintaining congenial socio-economic conditions of the fishing communities. Information on behavioral aspects such as level of awareness, attitudes, aspirations, motivation, impact of technology diffusion, etc. are significant for arriving at appropriate management decisions (Carole and Stone 1989). Information flow is an essential component for the success of any system or management scheme. It is also necessary for feedback and evaluation of project accomplishments.

Technology transfer requires firm linkages between research and extension. Technology is developed through research, and extensionists must have access to researchers' know how to ensure its successful transfer to fish farmers. Institutional linking of research and extension activities based on communication and information systems shall provide an organic link between them to contribute effectively. Research activities become ineffective and insignificant without feedback from fish farmers and fishers. Extension agencies shall lag behind in technological innovations if access to research information is not effective. Therefore, communication system should be open and multi-directional to ensure flow of information between policy-makers, scientists, extensionists, fishing communities and other stakeholders. A model that is dynamic and participatory is given in Figure 43.

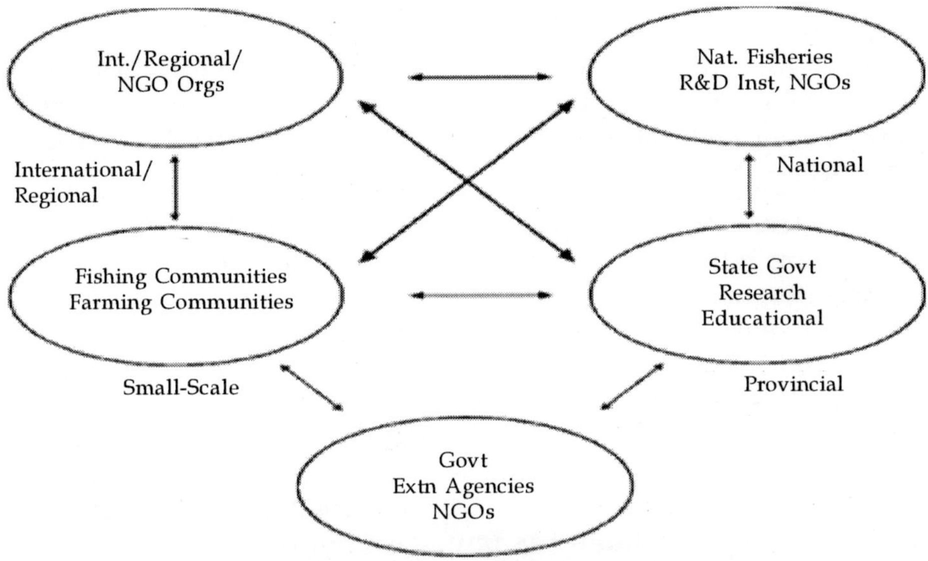

Figure 43. Model Information Flow in Fisheries Sector

Presently, gaps, deficiencies and barriers exist in the flow, dissemination and accessibility of fisheries information. Information capacity in terms of information services, access to relevant information and the skills required to participate in the global information services remains inadequate in the sector. The fisheries database and information resources are adequate but infirm in communication, dissemination and services. It needs further strengthening by application of ICT, notwithstanding the efforts made by several agencies. These resources are the stock-in-trade of state-funded libraries, research institutions and education institutions.

Trainings, printed materials and community intermediaries such as extension officers, NGOs, teachers, experienced fishers, etc. are the preferred sources of information for the fishers and the fish farmers. Internet also is a major resource for information. Measures to meet the information needs of small-scale fishing communities and fish farmers are inadequate and critical in the country. Stakeholders in the sector need skill development for accessing information effectively and efficiently for optimization of information generated in the sector.

The dissemination of fisheries information is the least developed field in the whole of agricultural information systems. Fisheries information is scattered between various government agencies, scientific and academic institutions and industry. Information access depends upon the person's experience and their influences in the sector. Need of information varies from research to trade, from subjects as diverse as biology, economics, nutrition, environmental science, and social and cultural norms. An efficient information system is absent in the sector that relates the needs of stakeholders.

Scientists and managers in the sector are to develop skills in using information retrieval systems designed with technology-prompted changes for the quality and timeliness in research, development, decision making, learning and teaching that affect the production of goods and services in the sector. Eugene Garfield, the famous information scientist, citation analyst and the founder of the Institute for Scientific Information (ISI), Philadelphia when asked by Istvan Hargittai about his dreams, said "I find it is very frustrating that so many scientists are ignorant of what they could do with information retrieval systems. I think it is important not only to be literature-minded, but to develop citation consciousness. I'm not sure how you teach this. It requires indoctrination by informed mentors".

❑❑❑

Chapter-8

Fisheries Informatics and Communication

Information and Communication Technologies (ICT), has paved way for dramatic developments in knowledge dissemination in all spheres of life and fisheries cannot be an exception. ICT enable universal access to information irrespective of physical location of content and information remains accessible 24 hrs 365 days. Libraries have always been the important tool for information transfer. By harnessing digital technologies, Library and information systems in fisheries sector can also usher in newer and innovative information services. The present chapter examines ICT based information transfer services and extension programmes in fisheries sector.

Role of ICT in Information Services

Current technologies facilitate processing and transfer of information by electronic means which includes everything from radio and television to telephones (fixed and mobile), computers and the Internet. In fisheries, ICT is used across the sector, from resource assessment, capture or culture to processing and commercialization. Some are specialist applications such as sonar for locating fish. Others are general purpose applications such as Global Positioning Systems (GPS) used for navigation and location finding, mobile phones for trading, information exchange and emergencies, radio programming with fishing communities and Web-based information and networking resources (FAO 2011). Considering importance of information as the critical input in the fisheries research and development, several value-added services have been launched to enhance connectivity and information transfer in India. The following sections survey some of the selected information services in agriculture, fisheries and related sectors in India.

Initiatives of ICAR

Fisheries education, research and development come under Indian Council of Agricultural Research (ICAR). Several ICT-driven information delivery mechanisms have been developed in the ICAR system for quick, reliable and cost-effective message delivery. ICAR provides e-linkage to 192 *Krishi Vigyan Kendras* (KVKs) and eight Zonal Project Directorates (ZPDs) located across the country to enable close and fruitful partnerships between the subject-matter specialists of the KVKs and the research scientists, extension-workers, fishers and fish farmers (ICAR 2012). ICAR website provides links to information on fisheries, agro-advisories, press releases, news updates, current events, journals and various national/international agricultural organizations/resources. The ICAR is the designated National Input Centre for Agricultural Research Information System (AGRIS) database of the Food and Agriculture Organization of the United Nations (FAO) since 1975 (Hasan 2012). Lately, a World-Bank-funded project on 'Mass Media as Message Multiplier' has been launched to utilize different modes of communication in an integrated manner for accelerated and sustainable delivery of messages. The Directorate of Knowledge Management in Agriculture (DKMA) delivers ICAR technologies, policies and products in print, electronic and web mode.

- **e-*Granth:*** e-Granth provides digital access to library resources of 12 different agricultural research institutions and agricultural universities which include OPAC, important institutional repositories, rare books and old journals and makes them publically accessible over internet under National Agricultural Research System (NARS) with Online Computer Library Center (OCLC) partnership. It has been developed to strengthen Digital Library and Information Management under the NARS. CIFE is the only fisheries institute under the group. *E-Granth* Open Access Repository of rare books and old journals is also planned for implementation (ICAR *e-Granth* 2013).
- ***KrishiPrabha:* Indian Agricultural Doctoral Dissertations Repository:** *KrishiPrabha* (e-Thesis) is the full-text, searchable and downloadable online electronic database of Indian agricultural doctoral dissertations submitted by research scholars to the State Agricultural Universities (SAUs) during the period 2000 to 2014. This database listing about 7900 doctoral theses with a full text of about 6250 Dissertations has been created by Nehru Library, Ch. Charan Singh Haryana Agricultural University, Hissar (Nehru Library 2014).

- **Consortium for e-Resources in Agriculture (CeRA):** Consortium for e-Resources in Agriculture (CeRA) provides online access to international journals related to agriculture and allied sciences from eight publishers to all the NARS libraries, SAUs and Colleges of Agriculture/Veterinary/Fisheries on 24hrs 365 days basis. It contains about 300 subscribed international/national journals in agriculture, fisheries and related subjects. About 35 foreign journals are specific to fisheries and related subjects. It also provides gateway access to 2000 online free e-journals (CeRA 2013).
- **Farmer Mobile Advisory (FMA):** Farmer Mobile Advisory (FMA) is an information delivery service on mobile phones. FMA technology provides an opportunity for sharing and exchanging knowledge more widely and in a more cost-effective way than was previously been possible. In the agricultural field where farmers are working in hard-to-reach and geographically spread areas, support can be provided by extension workers over the phone or by text instead of waiting for them to visit the region. Information about market prices and weather conditions can also enable farmers to make informed decisions about their crops (CABI 2013). Kissan Mobile Advisory (KVK-KMA), service for information delivery was launched in Karnataka in 2010. The programme envisages to advice farmers with need based information on every Tuesday and Friday by the KVKs (ICAR 2013).

Initiatives by Ministries/Departments, Government of India

Various Government Departments have launched services that aim to improve the reach of information to the stakeholders.

- **Agriculture Resources Information System Network (AGRISNET):** Agriculture Resources Information System Network (AGRISNET) is a mission mode project funded by the Ministry of Agriculture. It is in operation across the country, targeting state/district agricultural and allied departments to provide improved services to the farming communities. AGRISNET aims to develop comprehensive online knowledge portal to disseminate relevant information to farmers. The goal of the project is to follow an all-inclusive approach in terms of ensuring technological connectivity, development of system software and provision of hardware at agriculture department offices up to the block level in all states and union territories (Moni 2004).
- **Knowledge Help Extension Technology Initiative (KHETI):** KHETI is a participatory ICT solution experimented with rural poor

farmers, designed on mobile phone platform. One can create Short Dialogue Strips (SDSs) using six images and 1.5 minutes voices on their queries and problems. The KHETI system aims to speed-up and improve communications amongst various stakeholders especially between the co-operatives, agriculture specialists, farmer representatives and farmers (Rizvi and Dearden 2012).

- **Agricultural Marketing Information Network (AGMARKNET)**: Agricultural Marketing Information Network (AGMARKNET) is a G2C (G2C denote electronic sharing of data and information systems between government to citizen) e-governance portal that caters to the needs of various stakeholders such as farmers, industry, policy makers and academic and research institutions by providing agricultural marketing related information from a single window (Suri et al 2012). AGMARKNET, an initiative by the Union Ministry of Agriculture, links around 7,000 agricultural wholesale markets in India with the State Agricultural Marketing Boards and Directorates for effective information exchange. The e-governance portal implemented by National Informatics Centre (NIC) for AGMARKNET facilitates web-based dissemination of prices and commodity arrival information from agricultural produce markets to producers, consumers, traders, and policy makers transparently and quickly. The service is available in eight regional languages and in English (AGMARKNET 2013).

Similarly, the gateway to the Department of Agriculture and Cooperation (DAC) portal named DACNET connects DAC directorates and their field units. The portal provides information on agricultural statistics, production, economics, etc (DACNET 2013). The SEEDNET and the Plant Protection Informatics Network (PPIN) of the Central Insecticides Board and Registration Committee (CIBRC), available at http://seednet.gov.in provides information services on seed protection, certification, etc (CIBRC 2013). Web based Plant Quarantine Information System of Directorate of Plant Protection, Quarantine and Storage (DPPQS), available at http://plantquarantineindia.nin.in, provides information services on plant protection, quarantine and storage (DPPQS 2013). *E-Krishi, mKrishi, Ikisan*, etc. are other examples of ICT based services in the agriculture sector of India. *Gyandoot* Project (an Intranet in Dhar District Madhya Pradesh connecting rural cyber cafes catering to the everyday needs of the masses) and *Bhoomi* (project of on-line delivery and management of land records in Karnataka) are some of the other e-governance initiatives in India (ICAR 2010).

- ***Agropedia:*** *Agropedia* is an online knowledge repository for information related to agriculture, fisheries and other areas in India. It is one stop shop for information, pedagogic or practical knowledge related to extension service in Indian agriculture and, includes universal meta-models and localized content for a variety of users with appropriate interfaces built in collaborative mode in multiple languages. *Agropedia*, designated as 'agricultural Wikipedia' by IIT, Kanpur, is intended for open learning, sharing and empowering farmers by hosting wide range of agricultural information. *Agropedia* portal at http://agropedia.iitk.ac.in/ consists of a knowledge repository, a social networking platform and content distribution service that uses advanced web technologies and links web space to mobile telephony. Knowledge models (total 11) developed for *Agropedia* are used for tagging and searching repository objects. These models are universal and can be extended and adopted for any agro-climatic zone. By employing state-of-the-art practices and techniques of the semantic web, *Agropedia* enables specialists in the agriculture/fisheries research, education and others interested in these areas to contribute to the knowledge base. The users have a choice to contribute towards the *Gyan Dhara* (Certified Content) or to participate in the interaction space for contributing to *Jan Gyan* (Emergent Knowledge). Thus, the users of *Agropedia* are the architects of the knowledge, as well (*Agropedia* 2013).

Informatics led Services in India

National information networks and services useful to the fisheries sector are discussed in the following sections.

- **National Portal:** National Portal of India at ***india.gov.in*** has been developed with an objective to enable a single window access to information and services provided by the various Indian Government entities. The content in this Portal is the result of a collaborative effort of various Ministries and Departments at the Central/State/District level. This Portal is Mission Mode Project under the National e-Governance Plan, designed and maintained by NIC. The portal attempts to provide comprehensive, accurate, reliable and one-stop source of information about India and its various facets (Government of India 2013). Links are provided to other Government of India Portals and websites. Fisheries production statistics, resource statistics, export, plan outlays, etc. are also available in the Portal. The need for India's comprehensive statistical information is served by the portal at www.IndiaStat.com, providing recent, exhaustive, authentic socio-economic statistical analysis and yearly data statistics classification about agriculture, census, economy, education, etc.

- **Ocean State Forecast Services of INCOIS:** Ocean State Forecast (OSF) providing forecast of wave, swell and wind parameters for tropical Indian Ocean at six hourly intervals and forecast of tidal currents along the Indian coasts at three hourly intervals are generated and published daily on Indian National Centre for Ocean Information System (INCOIS) website. INCOIS disseminates coastal wave forecast through All India Radio (AIR) and FM stations along the Indian coast. The broadcast are given thrice a day for different locations. The information on wave height, wind speed and their directions are disseminated in local languages through AIR and other public addressing systems (INCOIS 2007). Coastal states have nodal centre for dissemination of OSF through AIR in the regional languages.
- **Potential Fishing Zone (PFZ) Advisory Services of INCOIS:** Potential Fishing Zone (PFZ) is a unique service wherein identification of potential fishing zones indicating the availability, type and quantity of fish is notified to the fishing communities for economical fishing activity. PFZ Advisory service is unique in terms of its multi lingual operability, frequency, innovation and novel way of dissemination. PFZ generated on every Monday, Wednesday and Friday are disseminated to about 500 fish landing centers/fishing villages over telephone, fax, e-mail, website, Doordarshan, All India Radio, news media and Electronic Display Boards (EDB), covering the entire coastline of India (INCOIS 2007). The web-based multi-lingual on-line information delivery system with Web-GIS capability enables the users to query, analyze, visualize and download ocean data, information and advisories for their regions of interest.
- **Registration and Licencing of Fishing Craft (ReALCraft):** 'ReALCraft' is a work-flow based online application system for Vessel Registration under Marine Fishing Regulation Act to the fishing vessels operating along the Indian coast. It is a national project sanctioned by the Department of Animal Husbandry, Dairying & Fisheries (DAHDF) for implementation in all coastal States and Union Territories (ReALCraft 2013). ReALCraft aims to bring all the Indian fishing vessels under one hub. The National database shall enable tracking of registered vessels at any point of time from anywhere, strengthen coastal security and security of fishermen in the sea, electronic issuance of registration, license certificates, etc.

Digital Repositories

The NARS has only two institutional repositories at present (1) Eprints@CMFRI, the digital repository of Central Marine Fisheries Research Institute (CMFRI) at http://eprints.cmfri.org.in/and (2) Eprints@IARI, the digital repository of Indian Agricultural Research Institute (IARI) at http://eprints.iari.res.in/. Eprints@CMFRI is the only Open Access repository in fisheries in whole of NARS. At present, creation of the repositories in NARS is largely individual efforts. The digital repository of National Institute of Oceanography (NIO) named DRS@nio at http://drs.nio.org attempts to collect, preserve and disseminate different institutional publications on oceanography and aquatic science (NIO 2013). National Information Centre for Marine Sciences (NICMAS) maximizes NIO library resource utilization. '*IndOcean*', database of abstracts on Indian Ocean literature which contains over 34000 records are made searchable online by NICMAS (NICMAS 2013). Digital repository of Ministry of Earth Sciences (MoES) named ePrints@MoES collects, preserves and disseminates the research output created by the MoES research community. ePrints@MoES repository is running on ePrints open archive software, a freely distributed archive system available from http://eprints.org. ePrints@MoES complies with the OAI framework allowing publications indexed by web search engines and other indexing services (MoES 2013). The Open Access Institutional Repository of Rajiv Gandhi Centre for Aquaculture Research (RGCA), ePrints@RGCA, contains RGCA generated journal papers, conference papers, reports, theses, patents, etc. self-archived by RGCA scientists (RGCA 2013). This repository is linked to ePrints@cmfri for search results.

National Knowledge Network (NKN)

National Knowledge Network (NKN), the Project of Government of India, is aimed at establishing a strong and robust internal Indian network, capable of providing a unified, secure and reliable backbone for managing knowledge resources in all the sectors. NKN also aims towards ushering in a knowledge revolution in the country with connectivity to more than 1500 institutions with the state-of-the-art pan-India network, facilitating the development of India's information infrastructure (NKN 2013). NKN has established Video Conferencing and Internet Protocol telephony facilities at select ICAR institutes connected on the ICAR- Education and Research Network (ERNET) network to facilitate real time communication. NKN has provided links to all the ICAR institutions and SAUs with 100 mbps broadband. NKN is beneficial in connecting all universities, libraries, laboratories, agricultural and fisheries institutions to share data and resources as NKN is congruent with e-Governance in the country. NKN provides platform rather than services. It is up to the institutions and agencies to utilize it for information management systems and services.

Strategies of ICT Based Information Services

A greater understanding of the information scenario should form the starting point for informatics led development in the sector. The author notes that the national agencies and institutions have not taken up fisheries informatics seriously in India. However, individual entrepreneurs and researchers are interested in discussing issues on innovative technologies in aquaculture and fisheries, but with less digital provisions. Strategies that need attention are discussed in the following sections.

Resource Sharing

The fisheries information system resources can be classified into (1) information resources, (2) infrastructure (3) manpower resources and (4) financial resources. It is noted that there are feeble activities on resource sharing and cooperation between information divisions and institutions in the sector. Some of the services discussed elsewhere are only non-starters or paper tigers. The feeble resource sharing activities in the sector are given in Table 10.

Table 10. Information Resource Sharing Activities in Fisheries Sector

Activity	Participants	Service	Benefit
Inter Library Loan	Nil	Nil	Nil
Union Cataloguing, etc.	CIFE	WorldCat	OCLC Membership
Member ship in JSTOR/ IAMSLIC/ ASFA, etc.	CIFT	ASFA input Centre	Free Access to ASFA database
Consortium on Journal Subscription	ICAR Inst/ SAUs/CoFs	CeRA	Access to journals included in CeRA
Digital Repository/ETD	CMFRI	eprint@cmfri	Open Access to documents/Theses
Library Training/ Orientation	Nil	Nil	Nil

Resource Sharing Programmes

The International Association of Aquaculture and Marine Science Libraries and Information Centres (IAMSLIC) is the association of individuals and organizations interested in library and information science, especially as these are applied to the recording, retrieval and dissemination of knowledge and information in all aspects of aquatic and marine sciences and their allied disciplines. The Z39.50 Distributed Library and Interlibrary Loan programme, with more than 90 member libraries from more than 25 countries is offering materials to other member libraries via interlibrary loan and document delivery (IAMSLIC 2013). Such resource sharing initiatives provide a helping hand to the organizations for exchange and exploration of ideas and issues of mutual concern. In India, NIO is the member of IAMSLIC.

Journal Storage (JSTOR), the international initiative for resource sharing has 411 member institutions from India, as on 04 Mar 2013. NIO is a member. Though many Indian universities and institutes are members, no fisheries institute is a member of JSTOR. From agriculture sector, Punjab Agricultural University is the only member. WorldCat, project of OCLC, enables libraries to connect to a larger world. Individual collections are linked together in a massive virtual collection that amplifies value for participating institutions and information seekers everywhere (Wikipedia 2013)

OCLC is a non-profit service and research organization that works consistently to lower information costs, identify issues and trends that impact the field, advocate the societal role of libraries and develop new technologies and standards that keep the libraries on the leading edge of technology. Connexion is OCLC's flagship cataloguing service and easy to use suite of tools with built-in access to WorldCat. Libraries use Connexion to create and edit quality bibliographic and authority records, to help users find the materials they need faster, and share records with the entire OCLC cooperative to the benefit of libraries around the world. CatExpress is a simple-to-use copy cataloguing tool. CatExpress can be used if the library needs basic copy cataloguing and MARC record delivery for 250-7000 titles per year. If the library catalogues more than 7000 titles per year, and/or needs to create original cataloguing records, Connexion is recommended by OCLC (OCLC 2012). Central Institute of Fisheries Education (CIFE) is a part of OCLC by participating in WorldCat programme.

Standards

The strength of the chain is in the weakest link. When resource sharing and ICT driven information dissemination systems are discussed, it is those standards that address technology-based product development and service provision that are of interest to the study on Fisheries Information. The ISO's standards definition stipulates that each standard contain specific criteria to be applied consistently to its respective function (Kochtanek and Matthews 2002). According to Deshmukh, (1990) standards ensure compatibility for networking of libraries and information centres in order to promote economy of human effort, cost and time, facilitate interchangeability of information across units of a network, improve the quality of information services and reduce the economic and technical barriers in information flow.

National Information Standards Organization (NISO) states that the standards relevant to library system and services are designed to achieve compatibility and therefore interoperability between equipment, data, practices, and procedures so that information can be made easily and universally available (NISO 2013). Thus, interoperability is the key to data retrieval and the standards make it possible to integrate hardware, software, and communications systems and to exchange information across boundaries of different systems (Radack 1990). Standards relating to information technology designs besides supporting interoperability are Bibliographic (Metadata), Communications, Search and Retrieve, and Markup.

AGROWEB-Digital Dissemination System for Indian Agricultural Research (ADDSIAR), an ICAR- National Agricultural Innovation Project (NAIP) funded project is aimed to identify standards, develop uniform guidelines, content management strategies and a model template for websites of ICAR institutes. Another ICAR project named E-publishing and Knowledge System in Agricultural Research (E-PKSAR) is aimed for electronic dissemination of information. Despite these projects, consensus on standardization for information sharing is not evolved in ICAR systems except adoption of template for websites of ICAR institutes. Jayasree and Subbiah (2000) in their study on bibliometric mapping of fisheries research in India have pointed out absence of subject descriptors, use of subject thesaurus, use of uniform field codes, etc. in database activities and recommended for uniform codes, standardization and common communication formats for interoperability and sharing of fisheries information sources. However, these aspects still remains a distant goal in the sector.

Resource Sharing Programmes in India

The success of Aquatic Science and Fisheries Abstracts (ASFA) is the adoption of common standards, formats and procedures among the participating centres in bibliographic records and information sharing. The main advantage of ASFA services are the quality, speed and good back-up. Ernest J Mann rightly observed that the model adopted by ASFA on organization, management, coordination and data processing; acts as a spring-board for any cooperative abstracting and indexing programme that could ultimately lead to the creation of a single, coordinated, world system for agricultural and food information (Mann 2014). Dr. Mann was one of the earliest scientists who contributed for the development of the subject 'Agricultural Informatics'.

The involvement of professionals and sectoral agencies in developing standards, uniform codes and communication formats is not encouraging. It is one of the major handicaps in information sharing capacity of the sector. Cloud Computing environment should emphatically and particularly be adopted in fisheries information sector for information management. A shift into the cloud mode shall be beneficial for the information systems because it has a lot of upsides in respect of cost, management, Information Technology (IT) resources, support, security, etc. Cloud Computing and, also Open Access philosophy infuse some sort of standardization in information management systems. Nevertheless, establishment of a national institution with clear mandates on all the above aspects only shall ensure information systems with barrier free information flow in the sector. Though ICAR and DAHDF are the premier agencies for fisheries development, they pay scant regard to Information/Documentation/ Library systems that catalyze KGEU in the sector. National fisheries institutions under these agencies do not have a structured library and information system.

Informatics led Services in Kerala State

There are a few initiatives in the agricultural sector of Kerala to improve the reach of the schemes and programs to the stakeholders.

- ***Kissan Kerala* (Karshaka Information Systems Services and Networking-Kerala):** *Kissan Kerala* is an integrated, ICT enabled multi-modal agricultural information system project of Department of Agriculture, Government of Kerala that provides several dynamic and useful information and advisory services for the farming community across the State (Coordinator *Kissan Kerala* 2011). The basic objective of the project is to provide 'Right Information to the Right Persons at the Right Time in the Right Place and in the Right Context' dynamically using a combination of delivery methods like advanced technology portal, television, Internet, telephone, and mobile phone by effective integration of ICT systems and tools. The farmers may choose any medium to seek the relevant information. Portal contains dynamic and static data of Production and Marketing support information for the farmers (Kissan Kerala 2013). Fisheries is not included in *Kissan Kerala*. However, fish farmers can post queries and they get answers. 'Agri Video' channel integrated in to the system contains many full-length videos on Fisheries. The project is an innovative one and helps officers, farmers and extension officers in improving efficiency, capacity and knowledge level as well.

- **Centre for E-Learning, Kerala Agricultural University (CEL KAU):** CEL KAU is an agri-infotech portal that provides knowledge on various aspects of crops, animal husbandry, fisheries, farm machinery, market prices, etc. by converting collection of technological queries asked by farmers. It provides reading Malayalam language also. CEL KAU pages aim to make local and frontier areas of farm technology available to the farmers and all other agri-stakeholders round the year, free of cost (CEL KAU 2013). It provides links to AGMARKNET, Vegetables and Fruits Promotion Council of Kerala's services on Market Prices, *E-Krishi* a market driven agri-initiative implemented by Kerala State IT Mission and Department of Agriculture.

- **FISHNET, Government of Kerala:** FISHNET, Government web service encompassing aspects of the socio-economic status of fishermen, fishing craft/gear, fishing resources, marine products export, social security, etc., is available at fishnetkerala.gov.in. FISHNET enables computerized registration and license issues of motorized, mechanized and non-mechanized fishing vessels. The alphanumeric registration numbers act as a key to all information regarding the vessel and its owner (The Hindu, National daily dated 12 Jan 2009). The web page lists the agencies entrusted with fisheries development, contact details of key officers besides giving an overall view of fisheries sector in Kerala. Nevertheless, this service is not updated with static information or dynamic information since then.

Access, Equity and Equality

Dr R.A. Mashelkar who played an important role in shaping India's science and technology policies, R&D Innovation, IPR, agricultural research system, etc. opined that in order to meet the twin objectives of growth with equity, knowledge cannot be the prerogative of a few; everyone in the society must have access to knowledge and should become a knowledge worker (Mashelkar 1999). Dr. M.S. Swaminathan, an advocate of sustainable development, in his dialog on Information Technology states that taking the benefits of new technologies to the economically and socially disadvantaged sections of the rural populations is a prerequisite for promoting a new paradigm of rural development based on concurrent and integrated attention to the imperatives of ecology, economics, employment, and equity (Swaminathan 1993).

According to M. Moni, a technocrat in the field of informatics and e-governance in the country, the developments in enabling technologies such as ICT, GIS Technology, GPS, and Supervisory Control And Data Acquisition (SCADA) facilitate 'Informatics Led Agricultural Development' which will be a step towards precision agriculture and enhancement of quality of life of the farming community in India. Informatics Led Agriculture Development will require a sophisticated ICT network, facilitating an integrated approach of 'Internet Technology' and sustainable 'Agriculture, Rural and backward Area Development' with its farm and non-farm linkages for sustainable livelihood of rural people (Moni 2004).

Dr V. Balaji (2010) Director, Technology and Knowledge Management, Commonwealth of Learning, Vancouver, BC, Canada, formerly Director of IT Divisions of ICRISAT, Hyderabad and MSSRF, Chennai, an expert in agricultural/fisheries information systems and networks, and a specialist in ICT applications to rural development, in an interview for this study opined that information systems and services have to be re-designed and re-modeled as per the needs of the stakeholders. Information services are to be brisk, timely and spreading, helping in managing disasters, outbreak of diseases and such eventualities. Mechanisms for filtering, validating and grading of information are also to be evolved. Magnitude of the spread of avian flu in Asia during 2010 has been quoted by him as an example for dissemination of accurate information with speed to the stakeholders. Validation process takes lot of time in India. He has recommended adoption of Open Distributed Technology Enhanced Learning (ODTEL) in Agricultural Informatics wherein the valid data are accepted by the user community and the rest rejected. Such system should be open to users contributing Certified Content or Emergent Knowledge by themselves which in turn shall provide quality resources and services. It was considered earlier that mass production shall affect quality and standard. But Japan has proved that the mass production can bring quality and standard in the products. It underpins the need of an information system that built in the lines of ODTEL that can result in to quality, need-based and location specific information services in fisheries sector.

Mr. B.K. Mishra (2011), Managing Director, FISHCOPFED in an interview stressed the need for fisheries information system linking various stakeholders ranging from fisheries institutions and academics to ordinary fishermen across the country to provide continuously updated and authentic data on fish prices and other fisheries information at various locations across the country. He also suggested for providing primary fishermen's cooperatives with computers and Internet access to link them with 220 fish landing centres. Though the measures suggested ensure reach of ICT to the grassroots, it needs a strong back up of informatics for deliverance of information services.

Dr A.P.J. Abdul Kalam (2011) former President of India proposed three types of connectivities - physical, electronic and knowledge - to motivate and enable the local population to create economic centres such as cold storages, fish processing, value addition, alternative employment oriented schemes during non-fishing days and those who are involved in capacity building of the fishing community. The physical connectivity refers to roads, jetties, landing centres; electronic to broadband fibre and wireless connectivity; and knowledge connectivity refers to transfer of knowledge by education and training by government.

These discussions endorse the view of Ernest J Mann's paper *Focus on Agricultural Information Transfer* published three decades ago and republished in *Informatics Studies* 1(1) Jan-Mar 2014 (Mann 2014). But national and international organizations and governments have failed to adopt strategies like the one Mann has suggested. Adopting his recommendations would have helped the world to have a better system for agricultural information dissemination than what we have now. Even after three decades, the crust of the suggestions advanced by Mann remains valid.

The effective utilization of ICT shall facilitate innovative and efficient information services, support management and provide cutting edge to the research programmes. It shall also provide sustainable fisheries, rural and backward area development with its farm and non-farm linkages. Cooperative endeavors in information and knowledge sharing shall also become feasible. Resource sharing increases effectiveness of information service systems. A wide range of technologies can be adapted and introduced so that the most remote communities and once appropriated by users, can have positive impacts on their lives. There are many challenges on the way of creation of rural ICT infrastructure, development of appropriate farmer-friendly content and maintenance of regular flow of information in an interactive mode. Informatics led services in operation now, mainly target the stakeholders of agriculture farming sector. Fisheries stakeholders largely remain unaddressed in such endeavours. Toll Free Helpline Call Centres, Kissan Mobile Messaging Service and other innovative and effective services should suitably be extended to fisheries sector also, after impact studies on such services in agriculture sector.

Digital archiving in the sector is very weak. It is noted that the Institutional wisdom, Grey Literature and Research Reports are poorly archived, leading to loss of historical and baseline information. Open Access philosophy is not well absorbed in the sector. Journal of the Marine Biological Association of India, accessible since 2007 is one sample of OA in the sector. There are poor opportunities and scarce resources to share, publish and disseminate the traditional knowledge, research findings and institutional wisdom. Visibility of the small-scale individual studies and findings is poor. ETDs in fisheries sector are very limited. Coverage of fisheries in *KrishiPrabha* is very limited. Eprints@cmfri, the only Digital Archival in fisheries sector has limited scope. Digital archiving of Indigenous/Traditional Knowledge is absent in the sector.

Need for a Fisheries Informatics Institute

The stark reality of the Agricultural Research Information System (ARIS) established under ICAR some 15 years back by spending millions of rupees and futile years without any results is a point to ponder. If ICAR has initially established a Central Institute of Agricultural Informatics entrusting the implementation of ARIS project, the agricultural sector would have seen magical transformation by now. Instead, project officers from different specializations with amateur or no knowledge in informatics handled ICT projects. Library and Information Professionals and informaticians were rarely associated with it or sidelined. ICAR could not even support some expert systems developed by visionaries in a few regions due to lack of vision, expertise and other reasons. Kerala Agricultural University which developed an information system and training facilities for Agricultural Informatics in the late nineties could not sustain those efforts due to incapacity of the decision makers at the helm of affairs. Even the in-house generated research information of SAUs and ICAR institutes were not digitized and made accessible. The huge ICT infrastructure developed using public fund has turned to be mere stack of computers and equipments. Agricultural information never flowed, stored or disseminated under ARIS and the physical infrastructure remained under utilized, and became obsolete even before they could think of putting information into them (Raman Nair 2012).

Therefore, an institution specializing in Fisheries Informatics is indeed in need to coordinate various information support systems meant for fisheries development in India. A specialized informatics institution with specified mandates shall be able to ensure implementation and development of a sustainable fisheries information system for the country. It is a preliminary requirement and priority before we embark on any information system development for fisheries. As the ICAR and DAHDF systems are not innate and realistic with the library/information/knowledge systems, an institution namely 'Central Institute of Fisheries Informatics' need to be established by Government of India as an independent institution with clear mandates and organizational hierarchy, under the Ministry of Agriculture. The institute shall give a strong back up for information services in all its diversity and complexity to the stakeholders of fisheries sector in India.

❑❑❑

Chapter-9

Fisheries Information System of India (FISI) : Conceptual Design and Development

India is rich in knowledge resources on fisheries. However, there are various constraints in the information cycle from creation, production, and dissemination to access for its effective use and sharing. These aspects have already been discussed in the previous chapters and it is felt that there is an urgency to ensure flow of information to all the stakeholders of fisheries sector. But, it is not easy to fulfill. The information used and produced by different stakeholder categories involved in fisheries are characterized by the breadth of subjects dealt, its historic depth, the scale from local to global and the diversity of information sources. UGC (1988) in its report on Development of an Information and Library Network has stated that in research and development, lessons learned are often lost because of inadequate opportunities to disseminate information with speed. Utilization and validation of what has already been achieved depend upon the effective dissemination, sharing and preservation.

Therefore, an Information System based on ICT and resource sharing only can address these problems prevailing in the sector. This chapter deals with Fisheries Information System of India by examining the aspects of design and development of an integrated fisheries information system and network for India. An attempt is also made to cover the system concept, objectives, functioning, organisation, implementation, etc. of Fisheries Information System of India (FISI), an institution for implementation of FISI (Central Institute of Fisheries Informatics-CIFI), network system of FISI (Fisheries Information System Network-FISNet) and National Fisheries Portal (NFP) with information service components that should go into NFP. Frameworks of an information system such as network model, network schema, information flow model, architecture, components, standards, procedures, formats, cloud computing, network backbone, partners, pre-requisites and execution aspects are also attempted. FISI is proposed as a hierarchy of sub-systems, interdisciplinary in nature and it seeks to integrate technological disciplines with Library and Information Science, Management and other disciplines such as, Computer Science, Electronics, Communication and Fisheries Science.

System Definition

According to Vickery and Vickery (1994), system definition is not easy. But a few who attempted, defined it as a regularly interacting or interdependent group of items forming a unified whole, an integrated assembly of interacting elements, to carry out co-operatively a predetermined function (Cleland and King 1969) and as a set of parts coordinated to accomplish a set of goals (Churchman 1968). According to Mingers and Stowell (1997) 'Information system' is the effective design, delivery, use and impact of information technology in organizations and society. Atherton (1977) defines information system from the functional point of view as an unique integration of men, methods, organizational patterns and software elements whose coordinated operations provide manifold dispersed communities of users with all the input data relevant to them at any time, irrespective of origin or physical location, in a variety of possible output formats selected by them as best suited to their information gathering habits, abilities and requirements. According to Devarajan and Kurien (2011) the information system is an organized procedure for collecting, processing, storing, and retrieving information to satisfy a variety of needs. It is conceived as a set of interrelated components that jointly switch information from procedures to users, following identical or compatible rules and procedures with a view for worldwide exchange and interconnections.

The present information scenario is far from satisfactory in spite of resources and infrastructure invested in the sector. Though enormous public funds are expended, a structured National Information System for fisheries is not operational in India. A comprehensive information base and services based on it are also not formed and operated. Limited services are dispersed over numerous institutions spread throughout the country. They are not coordinated and networked for information access. National policies and frameworks for information systems in the sector are limited and remain largely fragmented. This lacuna leads to ineffectual strategies in fisheries sector.

Fisheries Information System of India (FISI)

Institutions are fundamental to the economic change. Presently, information services by fisheries institutions in India do not satisfy the information needs of the stakeholders, especially farmers and the fishermen community at the grass root level though there are research and extension systems operative in the agricultural systems of Union and State governments. It is pertinent to implement fisheries information system to accelerate the productivity and efficiency of research, education, extension and development in fisheries sector of the country. The FISI established thus can overcome those serious constraints prevailing in the sector that prevent systematic access to information. The problem is mainly with access to information rather than resources. The resources in the present form are also difficult for use by the stakeholders from top managers to the grass root fish farmers. There is no integration, resource sharing, standards and protocols for dissemination of information in spite of investments for huge ICT infrastructures, and projects related to information and knowledge programmes launched by ICAR and other agencies. The proposed FISI consists of different institutions at different tiers as nodes of the system so as to enable integration of resources and methods.

Objectives of the FISI

Bernus, Mertins and Schmidt (2006) says that an information system is a system for collecting, processing, storing, retrieving, customizing and distributing information within the enterprise and between the enterprise and its environment. The information system is a functionally defined subsystem of the enterprise, i.e. it is defined through the services it renders. Accordingly, the FISI is envisioned to provide and maintain an integrated information flow throughout the sector, so that right information is served whenever and wherever needed, in the quality and quantity needed and in the format that is familiar to the user. The objectives of the FISI are:-

1. To build an efficient information management and dissemination system that could reach fish farmers, fishers, public research institutions, administrators and entrepreneurs, which will be

accessible anywhere at any time by all concerned, which constantly updates content and technology, introduces new technology and services where in rural community can have more access.

2. To function as a network to aggregate, share and disseminate information of importance and interest to the fish farmers, fishers, entrepreneurs and officials in ways that enhance development of the sector.
3. To provide a fisheries information system platform that integrate the core competencies of partner institutions, enabling joint design, development, cost effective products and marketing of the knowledge products.
4. To develop uniform hardware and software for use of participating organization and the professionals and executives in the sector.
5. To provide a model and assist in developing fisheries information system in the States of India suiting to the local requirements.
6. To formulate and implement standards for processing and sharing of information online and offline that goes hand in hand with international standards adopted by FAO and other agencies for information sharing.
7. To assist and cooperate in the works of national agencies towards creation of Common National Information Infrastructure and 'Clouds' over a period of time that provide ready-to-use and secure environments for computing operations as well as users.
8. To build common service delivery platforms in association with the agencies of Common National Information Infrastructure.
9. To support directly or through participation the regional fisheries organizations and similar international information systems to benefit mutually in national, regional and international programmes for information exchange and dissemination.

Implementation

Dissemination of information is essential for empowering fisheries sector wherein the major stakeholders are rural communities. Communication is central to this process. The present day technologies are capable for the efficient response to the information needs of the users. The sectoral users mainly constituting rural communities need information related to fish farming, health, micro credit, government services, employment opportunities, training, education, support in production, storage and marketing of farm products, etc. Therefore, Web based information services mainly as Portal is suitable for FISI.

The FISI can be implemented on mission mode. Central Government has to provide funds. The programme should be executable as per specific proposals submitted by a Working Group comprising of experts from concerned fields. Fisheries libraries of National/State levels for Research/Education/Extension shall be the nodal centres of the system network. The initial cost for the physical (civil) infrastructure at central and nodal centres such as premises, site preparation, furniture, etc. should be met from central funds.

Central Institute of Fisheries Informatics (CIFI)

The FISI will be a decentralized system with centralized coordination and control by the Central Institute of Fisheries Informatics (CIFI). The CIFI will have clear mandates and shall be assigned with responsibility for implementation, functioning and development of the FISI.

Objectives of the CIFI

1. To establish systems and facilities in the country to provide services, appropriation of information and to meet user needs for sound and effective fishery science/management decisions.
2. To create awareness among all stakeholders, developing specific knowledge, market and trade information, advisory and decision support, offering short term training programmes, etc. through its consortium partners.
3. To function as a platform for dissemination of fisheries information by building portals, digital repositories and gateway functions.
4. To establish and coordinate resource sharing mechanisms by avoiding duplication of efforts, resources and services in the sector.
5. To update technologies, introduce services, invent vehicles for information exchange and innovate information products on a constant basis by duly considering the expertise and experience of other agencies functioning on similar sector/subjects/fields.
6. To promote research, development and innovation on regular basis in fisheries information transfer to meet the needs of the stakeholders.

7. To build and integrate State and Central systems to improve data management/ data access facilities, capable of supporting timely delivery of information to users in fisheries sector.
8. To promote national, regional and international cooperation and liaison for exchange of fisheries and aquatic science related information.
9. To establish national standards, policies, and best practices for data collection, management and dissemination, ensuring quality.
10. To provide training in all aspects of information and knowledge management to the LIS professionals in FISNet.
11. To leverage investments and to promote efficient use of resources across the country.
12. To maintain and publish a comprehensive inventory of information assets in authoritative databases.
13. To build and sustain effective partnerships to support collaboration among institutions/ stakeholders.

In order to fulfill above objectives, an apex body, namely the Central Institute of Fisheries Informatics need to be established by Government of India. CIFI shall be a high-level central focal agency for developing fisheries information system in the country, headed by a top-ranking official. CIFI should be given with inputs relating to information, man-power and expertise, facilities, building and equipments. CIFI shall have an executive authority, functional organization, costing and budgeting, operational capability, and infrastructure to function. CIFI shall rely on a multidisciplinary management team, including scientists from fisheries, library and information professionals, computer professionals, information and communication specialists, language technology experts and statisticians. CIFI can be located with NFDB, Hyderabad during initial years.

Organization of the CIFI

The organizational structure of CIFI proposed is on the functional basis. The organizational set up of CIFI with positions, committees and groups for the management, functions and services is given in Figure 44.

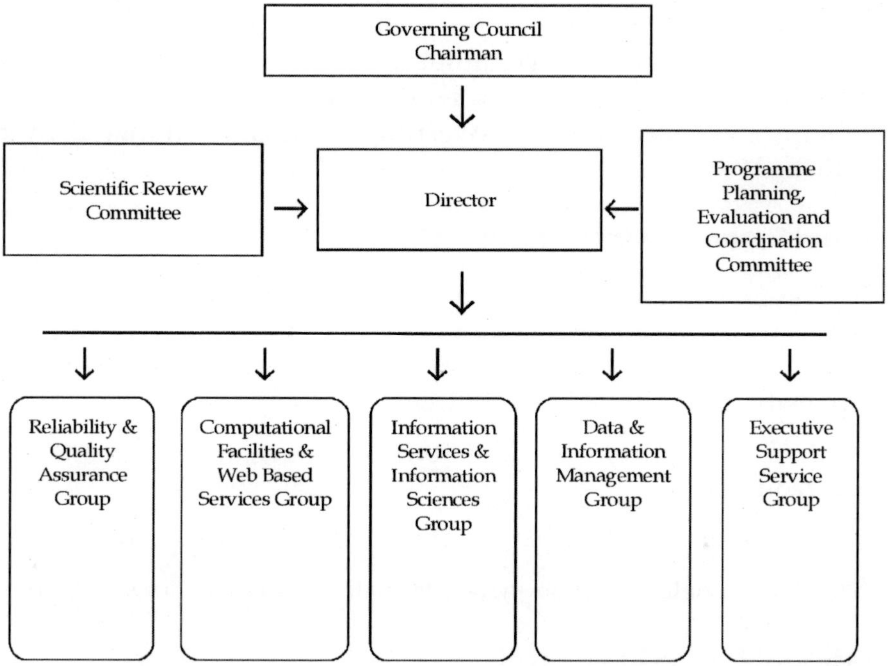

Figure 44. Organization Structure of CIFI

The CIFI will have a Governing Council, and its members may consists of the Director, National Informatics Centre (NIC); Programme Director, Directorate of Knowledge Management in Agriculture (DKMA), ICAR; Head, Department of Computer Science and Engineering, Indian Institute of Technology (IIT) Kanpur; Librarian, National Information Centre for Marine Sciences, (NICMAS), National Institute of Oceanography (NIO); Programme Director, Information Education and Communication, MS Swaminathan Research Foundation (MSSRF); Joint Secretary (Fisheries), Department of Animal Husbandry, Dairying & Fisheries (DAHDF), Ministry of Agriculture and Director, Indian Institute of Information Technology and Management, Kerala (IITM-K). The Chairman shall be appointed by the Government of India on the grounds of his/her expertise, contributions and services in the field of information technology, networking, and library and information science. The CIFI will have a Director for programme planning and execution as executive head. The Director should be appointed from among the experts in the fields of communication, networking, library and information systems, by the Government of India on the recommendations of a select committee constituted by the Union Public Service Commission (UPSC). Expert groups as shown in the Figure 44 will be responsible for the span of activities concerned. Two committees of review and evaluation shall advice the Director. Chairpersons of these two committees shall be the subject experts in the Governing Council, nominated by the Chairman.

Nodal Fisheries Information Centres

The functional basis of the FISI shall be the Information Centres of the specialized institutions in the sector. They shall constitute the second tier in the system for functional responsibilities. Functional responsibilities of the Nodal centres are to:

- Select, acquire, store and retrieve information in response to requests;
- Announce, abstract, extract, index, collate information and
- Disseminate information in anticipation and in response to requests.

National Fisheries Portal

Creation and management of Indian Fisheries Portal is one of the functions of the CIFI. The CIFI shall have a National Fisheries Portal Content Management Team that shall examine all aspects of Content Contribution, Approval, Review and Archiving of information. The portal shall have static and dynamic information contents, multi language interfaces with an endeavor to continue the enhancement and enrichment of the Portal in terms of content coverage, design and technology on a regular basis. National Portal of India at india.gov.in shall be the model for the execution, operations and content contribution. The mother portal of the CIFI shall be the platform for inter nodal interaction. The portal designed and organized to provide easy access to the multitude of fisheries related information available within the FISI is envisaged to be the one-stop option for fisheries information and gateway.

Components of Information Services

The information service components proposed under the FISI are given below. Servicing, management and maintenance may be done at different locations. The list is not intended to stuff the Portal with information but to enlist vivid resources, demands and services to be considered for inclusion.

1. **Bibliographic Database:** Record of bibliographic reference to fisheries research and management.
2. **Document Database:** Digital repository of documents on fisheries studies, laws and policies.
3. **Fisheries Statistics:** Catch and effort information, time series data on landed and on-board catches and their corresponding effort units.
4. **Fisherfolk Database**: Census data of fisherfolk.
5. **Expert's Database**: Fisheries experts' information, contact details, etc.
6. **Fish Information**: Production, sources, culture methods, catch methods, technology, market price, etc.
7. **Fish Health and Disaster Management:** Fish diseases, prevention, cure, management of disasters/diseases.
8. **Communication and Extension:** Extension activities and related resources, audio, video, etc.
9. **Education Information:** Information on fisheries education institutions and their information resources.
10. **Management Information:** Policies, regulations, conventions, treaties and legislations.
11. **Export and Quality Control**: Fish inspection, quality control, food safety and other related information.
12. **Geographic Information:** Maps, observation systems and tools for analysis.
13. **Fisheries Licensing**: Rules and procedures of licensing process.
14. **Decision Support**: Interactive system for managers.
15. **Resource and Ecological Assessment**: Resource protection, conservation and associated ecological elements.
16. **Socio-Economic Assessment:** Demographic profiles, fishing activities, income and livelihood.
17. **E-services:** e-mail, chat, search, FAQs, archival, knowledge base, form processing, feed backs, etc.
18. **Virtual Krishi Vigyan Kendra**: E-Learning/extension/open/distance learning.
19. **Advisory Services:** Meteorological, market intelligence, etc.
20. **News:** Local, meetings, conferences and workshops calendar, regional initiatives and projects.

21. **Hyper Links to Online Resources:** Virtual Libraries, online journals, e-Repositories, global databases, resource centres, organizations, institutions, training and educational resources.

Fisheries Information System Network (FISNet)

Network is a set of inter-related Information Centres and systems associated with communication facilities, which are cooperating through more or less formal and institutional agreements, in order to jointly implement information handling operations with a view to pooling their resources for serving the users in an effective manner (Anderson with Minasi 1999). The FISI shall consist of components and processes, resources and system that deliver information products. The resources consist of network, software, hardware, data and human resources. The model of Information System Resources and Processes of FISI is given in Figure 45.

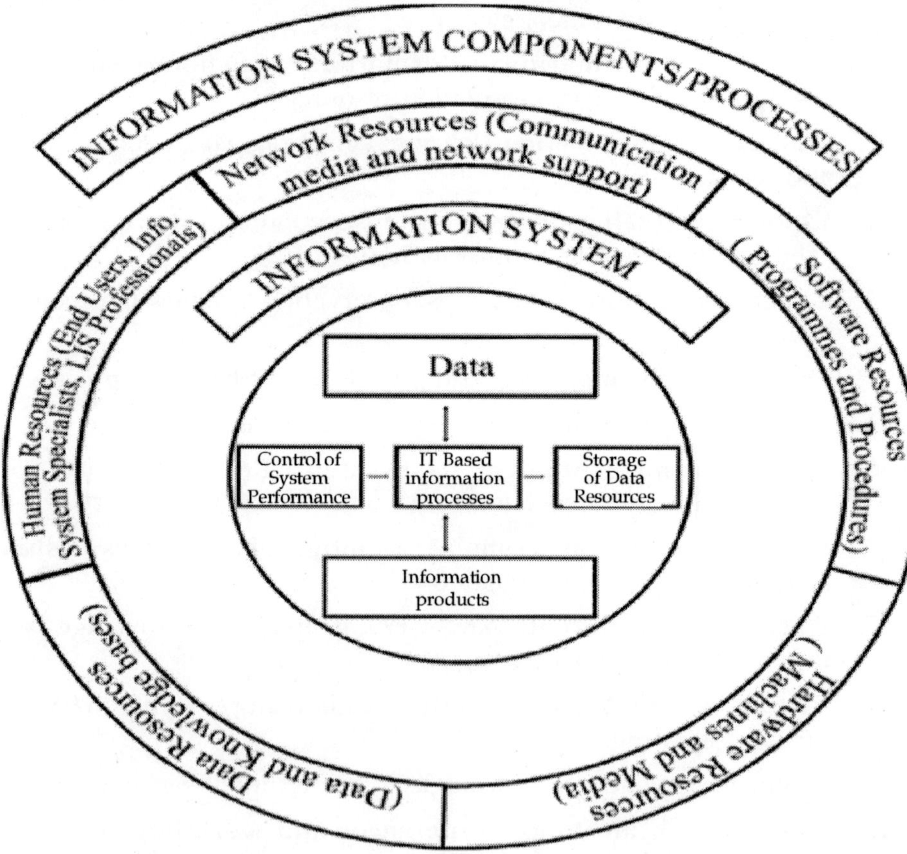

Figure 45. Information System Resources and Processes in FISI

The FISNet shall be the network frame of the FISI. The model of Network Schema of FISNet is given in Figure 46. Internet shall be the connecting medium for communication between member institutions. The component networks can exploit numerous telecommunication technologies, ranging from the dial-up telephone network to state-of-the-art broadband switching technologies. The FISNet model that ensures multi-directional, participatory, speedy and dynamic flow of Information and Knowledge is given in Figure 47.

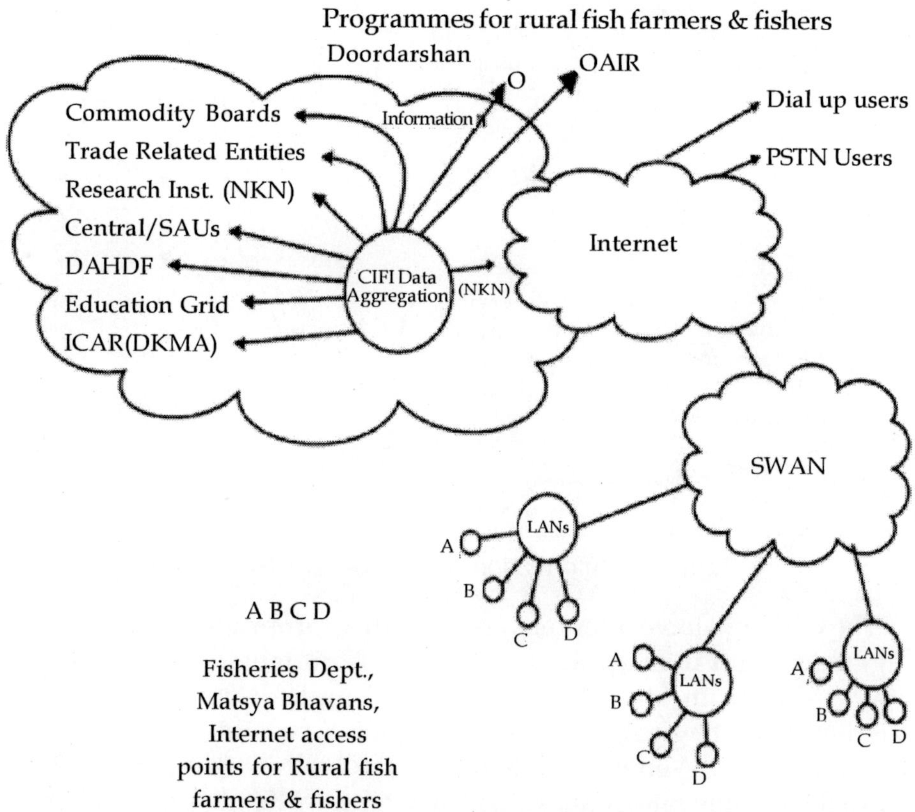

Figure 46. Network Schema of FISNet

State Wide Area Network (SWAN), the main connecting channel between the different Departments, provides a dedicated speedy channel for the efficient functioning of the e-governance applications. SWAN infrastructure that reaches even remote regions of the State shall be used by the FISI to implement network services and e-governance applications to the bottom line users. SWANs are integrated using National Knowledge Network (NKN) and envisaged as the converged backbone network for data, voice and video communications throughout a State (Jayakrishnan 2013).

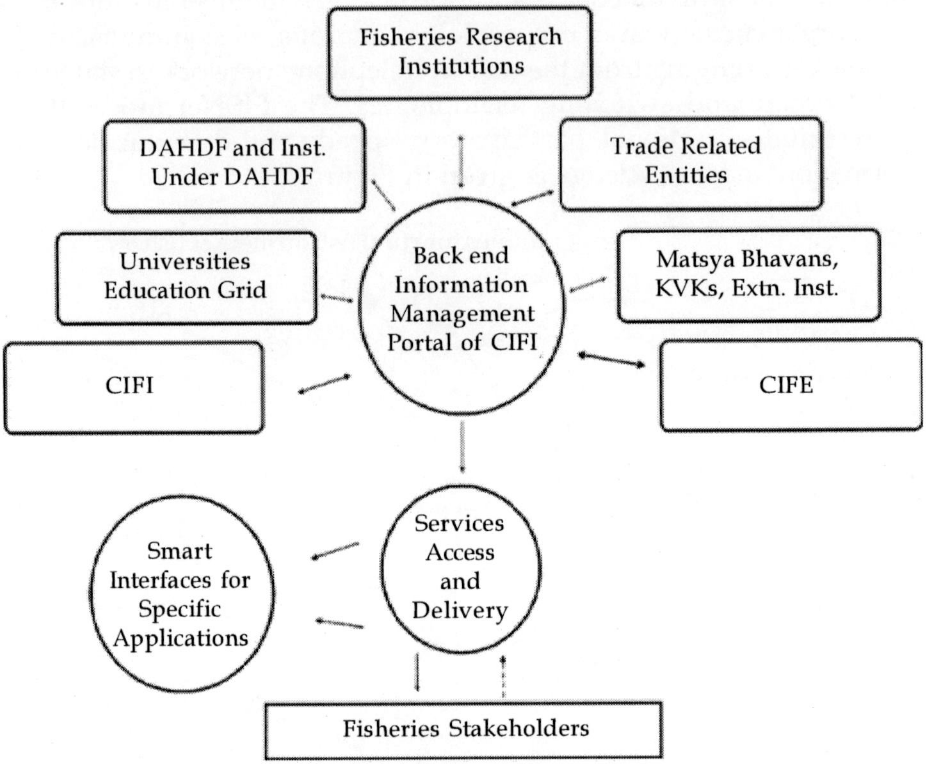

Figure 47. Information Flow Model of FISNet

The CIFI will have a server system with appropriate configuration to aggregate and manage all data coming from member institutions, for accessing from any part of the world and for content creation initiatives like Digital Libraries, Internet accessible Institutional Repositories, etc. Web server shall host the website of the CIFI. The CIFI shall facilitate information sharing over the FISNet. Various kinds of documents can be converted into HTML and made web-accessible. Policy papers, procedures, forms, annual reports, manuals, schedules, calendar of events, etc. can be converted to digital format and made accessible over the network.

Framework of the FISNet

Generally, a system framework needs to be developed by analyzing the basic functional processes of the System. The FISNet framework is envisaged with System Architecture and Technology Architecture. The System Architecture identifies the major modules of the systems network required to support FISI, the type of information maintained by each system module and the information flow between various modules and the Technology Architecture identifies the appropriate technology choices for the hardware and software to set up various modules. The network shall consist of: Core using Internet Protocol (IP) and Multi-Packet Labeled Services (MPLS) technology, an aggregation or distribution network, and an access or edge network linking the Local Area Network (LAN) of nodal centres to the core.

Model System Architecture

The model System Architecture of the FISNet is given in Figure 48.

Primary Framework and Principles

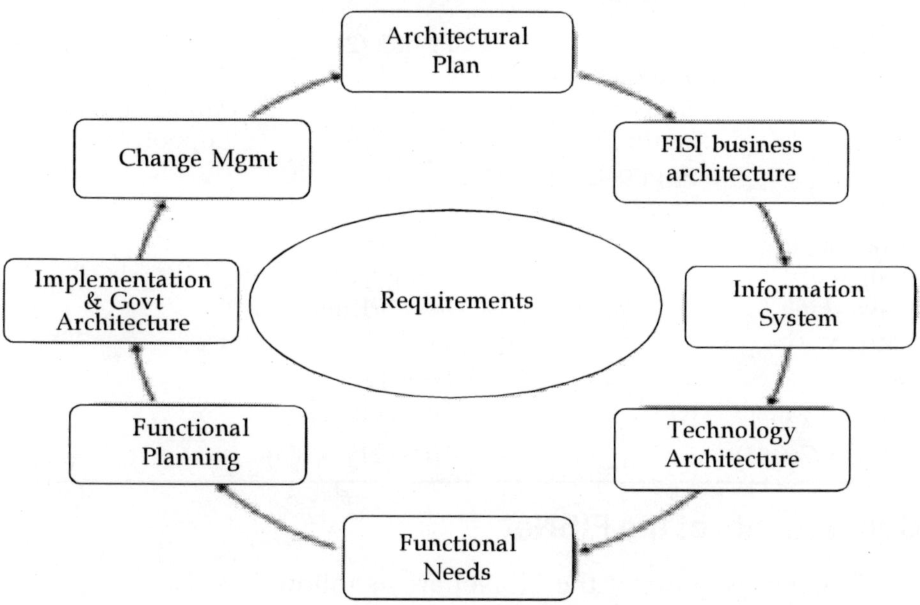

Figure 48. Model System Architecture of FISNet

Hardware and software requirements in approximates are given in Table 11. As technology is always in a flux, software and hardware choices proposed for the FISNet are not final. Software and hardware technology should be state-of-the-art at all times.

Table 11. Network Components of FISNet

Central		Nodal	
Hardware/ Networking components	**Software tools**	**Hardware/ Networking components**	**Software tools**
High Availability Servers (lower end) +OS (3) (Data base Server, Application Server, Patch/ Anti-virus Server)	Operating System for Server-(3)/OS for client (3) media+Firewall	High Availability Servers (lower end) + OS (2) (Database server and application server)	Operating System for Server (2)/ OS for Client (2) media +Firewall
Multi-media Clients (P-V or above) System+ OS (3)	Database Software and other access software tools including data security	Multi-media PC Client System+OS (2)	Database Software and other access software tools including data Security
Printers (3)	Office Productivity Tools with multi-lingual support	Printer (2)	Office Productivity Tools and Multilingual Support (2)
LAN infrastructure along with Networking interface	Development Kit	LAN infrastructure along with network interface	-
High End Scanners (3)	–	High End Scanners (2)	-
UPS (24x7x365)	-	UPS (24x7x365)	-

Components of the FISNet

The components of the FISNet are as follows:-

- Apex Centre : One (CIFI)
- Nodes : 10 (Fisheries Information Centres (in the first phase))
- Jurisdictions : 36 (29 Indian States and 7 UTs)
- Development Teams : Six (Project Committee and Divisions of CIFI)

- Support Centres : Two (NIC/NKN and ICAR (DKMA))
- Web Tools/Portals consisting of National Portal for Public view of fishery data, Provincial Portals and Themed Portals viz., Fish Genetic resources, etc.

State Department of Fisheries shall avail the State Data Centre (SDC) facility of the Government to host Web portal, digital library, union catalogue and databases required for its e-governance for fisheries stakeholders. SDC, the core component of the e-Governance infrastructure, consolidates services, applications and infrastructure to provide efficient electronic delivery of G2G, G2C, G2B and G2F services. (These acronyms denote electronic sharing of data and information systems between government agencies, departments or organizations: G2G government to citizen, G2C government to business G2B, G2F government to farmers). These services are rendered by the States through common delivery platform supported by core Connectivity Infrastructure such as SWAN and Common Service Centre (CSC) connectivity extended up to village level. State Data Centers provide functionalities like Central Repository of the State, Secure Data Storage, Online Delivery of Services, Citizen Information/ Services Portal, State Intranet Portal, Disaster Recovery, Remote Management and Service Integration by providing better operation and management control and minimizing overall cost of Data Management, and IT Resource Management. SDC acts as a mediator and convergence point between open unsecured public domain and sensitive government environment and enables various State Departments to host their services/applications on a common infrastructure (Jayakrishnan 2013).

Network Topology

A computer network topology is the physical communication scheme used by the connected devices. Common topologies include bus, ring, star and mesh. Network topology of the FISNet will be hybrid. The mesh topology of the NKN shall be the backbone network of the FISNet. Connectivity shall be provided by the NIC, the operating agency of the NKN.

National Knowledge Network (NKN)

NKN is the state-of-the-art pan-India network enabling to provide a unified backbone network for all the sectors and it is a critical information infrastructure for India to evolve as a knowledge society. It also facilitates integration of different sectoral networks in the field of research, education, health, commerce and governance. Backbone network ranges from 2.5 Gbps onto 10 Gbps connectivity between seven Supercore fully meshed locations pan India. The network is further spread out through 26 Core locations with multiple of 2.5/10 Gbps partially meshed connectivity with Supercore locations. The distribution layer connects entire country to the core of the network using multiple links at speeds of 2.5/10 Gbps. The end users are connected up to a speed of 1 Gbps. NKN is fully owned by Central Government. Therefore, NKN is recommended for FISNet, considering also (1) the enhanced connectivity with Ultra high speed network (2) facilitate information infrastructure without going into its complexities by edge institutions (3) single infrastructure that support multitude of applications in a secure manner and (4) scalable, adaptable and available on 24 x 7 x 365 basis.

Standards, Formats and Procedures

The CIFI shall implement standards and uniform guidelines in techniques, methods, procedures, hardware and software for communication, exchange and inter-operability of data, information and services. The library and information system standards shall be:

- Machine-Readable Cataloging MARC 21
- Anglo-American Cataloguing Rules (AACR)-II
- Open Archives Initiative-Protocol for Metadata Harvesting (OAI-PMH)
- Search/Retrieve URL-Search/Retrieve Web (SRU-SRW) Service
- NISO Circulation Interchange Protocol (NCIP) Z39. 83 Ver 2.0
- International Organization for Standardization (ISO) 2709
- Unicode 4.0 / 5.0
- Z39.50
- Code 39 [barcode]
- Fedora Digital Object
- Open Uniform Resource Locator, etc.

These Standards are expected to permit:

- Multi-tasking facility and customizable search
- Union Catalogue facility
- Simple and clear interface in English and other national languages
- Integration with email applications
- Unicode support for all languages
- Ability to integrate with various web 2.0 tools, RSS feeds, and similar plug-ins
- Multiple level admin/user logins and permissions settings
- User access management
- Backup and restore functionalities
- Automatic multilingual transliteration facility for search, retrieval and data entry
- Ability to handle multimedia and digital resources [MARC Tag 856] and
- Reports and ability to save reports in PDF, Word, Excel formats.

Cloud Computing

Cloud Computing is services and storage space sold and delivered over the Internet which has become a feasible model for organizations and institutions. Fisheries institutions may decide to cooperate and interconnect their computing infrastructure and create a community 'Cloud' which may be accessed by any of its members. Library/Information/content management systems can switch over to this facility to get networked storage facilities and various computer applications. Clouds relieve the participants from investing on huge infrastructures. Cloud Computing tends to adopt certain standards for information sharing, access and dissemination. Information centres can work as a system on common platform, integrate resources for maximum utility such as e-resources, processing, Union Catalogue, Digital Library, repositories and other value added services. CIFI shall have a strategy on how to make best use of cloud facility and function as a facilitating centre for Infrastructure-as-a-Service (IaaS) Cloud. The strategy shall amplify the power of cooperation in FISNet and maintain quality and standards of information services and products.

Participative Development

The FISI can provide the 'Knowledge and Interaction Hub for Indian Fisheries'. Virtual Krishi Vigyan Kendras *(vKVKs)* can be one of the main service modules of FISI. The knowledge repository, social networking platform and content distribution services in fisheries may adopt the frame work of *Agropedia,* with necessary changes in tags and information service categories in order to save efforts, cost and time. The resultant system can be termed '*Fishpedia*'. FISI can also take lead roles in introducing fisheries information services in line with *Kissan Kerala* in all the Indian States. 'Fishpedia' can be further developed with local participation as envisaged in *Agropedia.* In *Agropedia, Gyan Dhara* (Certified Content) and *Jan Gyan* (Emergent Knowledge) are the two modules that contribute to its knowledge base. *Jan Gyan* enables the concepts of Open Distributed Technology Enhanced Learning (ODTEL) in Information Systems.

Radio and TV

It is necessary that widely dispersed, digital information deprived stakeholders be given information they need through mass communication media such as radio and TV. Quality information processed and packaged by CIFI on best practices, farming and fisheries events, useful tips, new concepts, schemes, programmes, success stories, market prices and its analysis, weather information, advisory information, seasonal advisory information and a variety of SDI of value to the farmers and general citizens can be transferred to Doordarshan and AIR for telecast and broadcast.

Partners for Information and Network Services

As no single organization would be able to meet the aims of the FISI, many organizations are to be involved in the FISNet to serve fisheries stakeholders. Some of the organizations have already been referred to. The following list is not exhaustive, but is rather intended to identify organizations that are likely to have some role in the process.

- National Informatics Centre Network (NICNET)
- NKN and NIC
- National Fisheries Development Board (NFDB)
- ICAR (DKMA)

- Indian Institute of Information Technology and Management- (from States, with relevant contribution)
- Projects for ICT Application in different States like Information Kerala Mission (IKM)
- Select IITs
- DAHDF, Min. Of Agriculture
- State/UT Fisheries Departments
- MSSRF/NGOs
- Marine Products Export Development Authority (MPEDA)
- Doordarsan and
- All India Radio

These are some of the main stream and out stream institutions that can jointly perform. For example, CIFI and NIC can jointly form a Project Committee consisting of project executives from both the NIC (Technical) and the CIFI (Fisheries and Information Science) and also members from the partners. The Project Committee can suggest patterns for improving the system.

Pre-requisites

The CIFI can moot Agreements and Memorandum of Understanding (MoU) between the partners, agencies and providers of infrastructure and services. The CIFI can also ensure (1) Establishment of facilities and infrastructure for the network (2) Formulation of schemes for information services (3) Methods for delivery of information to users (4) Ensuring compatibility and interoperability for resource sharing and (5) Standardization of policies, procedures, formats and methods.

Execution

The FISI has to be structured along functional rather than organizational lines. The FISI shall be a three tier system consisting of Central Institute of Fisheries Informatics at the apex, Fisheries Information Centres as nodal points and Service Centres such as Village Knowledge Centres (VKCs), Village Information Centres (VICs), *Matsya Bhavans*, Fisheries Department Office, Extension Offices and NGOs at the grassroots. The FISI can be implemented in a phased manner. The first phase shall cover all the National fisheries institution libraries/information divisions that function as specialized divisions, traditionally collecting and disseminating records of fisheries science and of scientific thinking. At present, these divisions/libraries are not evolved in to Information Centres having innovative services, resource sharing and networking in fisheries sector. These libraries/divisions are to be modified as Fisheries Information Centres to commensurate with the objectives and aims of the FISI.

Libraries/information divisions attached to the National fisheries institutions are to be designated as the Library and Information Centre in that specialized field of the parent institution and shall form the specialized centre in the information system. For example, Central Institute of Brackishwater Aquaculture (CIBA) library can be designated as Brackishwater Aquaculture Library and Information Centre and shall form the specialized information centre in Brackishwater Aquaculture. The CIFI shall outline the models for the regional and sectoral nodal centres, the professionals, standards, protocols, services, etc. common for FISI. Signed agreements may be executed wherever required for implementation of network activities. Central funds shall be utilized for ICT infrastructure. The Information Centres shall be headed by Library and Information Science (LIS) professional of scientist level supported by computer and communication technicians, and LIS professionals as the services of the information system depends on the products of well-organized professionally staffed Information Centres.

In the second phase, national fisheries institutions that are deficient with library services such as FSI are to be up-graded with resources, services, professionals and hooked to the network. The CIFI can also implement State level information centres in consultation with respective State Government Departments. In the third phase, out stream institutions, universities and educational institutions engaged in aquatic, fisheries and fisheries related education and research are to be added to the FISI. Solutions on connectivity to the last mile service points such as VKCs, VICs, Matsya Bhavans, NGOs and Extension Offices shall be provided by the NKN. Solutions on information service provisions shall be dealt by the State government by establishing VKCs/VICs in Matsya Bhavans, Department Offices to facilitate knowledge services to the rural community stakeholders.

Factors for the Success

The factors for the success of the system implementation are maximally incorporated in the schema of FISI. It would require re-organization and re-alignment of the roles and responsibilities of related institutions and their relationships to the line ministries/ departments/agencies. The changes would need government support at the highest levels to ensure smooth completion of the processes. A phased and gradual implementation and development of FISI would allow a wider appreciation from the stakeholders of fisheries sector. Project planning techniques should be further explored to design, implement, and monitor the FISI and project management responsibilities should be clearly identified. To ensure easy absorption of the system by organizations, three phased implementation is suggested for FISI. Implementation of an integrated network is complex in a multi-agency environment. Cooperation between the agencies involved is necessary for the success of the system. FISI system design envisages a steering group with representatives from all major participant agencies to ensure the needs of all participant agencies. The lead responsibility for the different component modules of the overall system should rest with CIFI. As the organizational capacity of the agency of implementation is important, restructuring the organizational set up, upgrades of the status and levels of information professionals, salary upgrades for key posts, hiring of project implementation specialists, management specialists and other technical skills are to be addressed by CIFI from time to time.

An ongoing policy of training is inbuilt in FISI. Beside formal training programmes, the FISI design scheme facilitates for appropriate change management procedures so that staff shall feel comfortable in their new work environment. Relative authority and power relationship of individuals and groups within organizations are areas that need re-definition in the system. Information system support is distributed among several agencies in FISI. Therefore, mechanism for coordination among agencies is incorporated in the scheme so that a common set of policies, procedures, and standards are adopted in the system. It covers the protocols for communications, data entry, editing and updating, back-up and recovery, security, contingency and disaster plans, and technical and user documentation. The NKN/ NIC shall provide local presence, training and technical support for FISI.

Catalyzing Effect of ICT for Fisheries Development

Information system has the potential for improving the efficiency and effectiveness of research, education and extension in the sector. With regard to the primary stakeholders, it needs to be emphasized that the constraints in the sector cannot be fully solved using ICT and digital technologies. Nevertheless, ICT can contribute for their development. The proposals outlined here are preliminary and a detailed technical examination may be necessary, considering the complexity of the subject.

❑❑❑

Chapter-10

Agenda for National Planning and Implementation of FISI

An attempt is made in this chapter to outline an agenda for a national outlook on fisheries information sector. The implementation of the agenda will depend on actions taken at national and local levels and attention focused to make transformative shifts which can advance human and sustainable development that fisheries sector requires.

Information Sector

Information systems are omnipresent in the sector. However, it needs further strengthening by application of ICT, notwithstanding the efforts made by several existing agencies. The fisheries information resources are adequate but infirm in communication, dissemination and services. To a large extent, information gathering and utilization capacities are weak in the sector. Information capacity in the R&D system is somewhat better but information access capability at the grass root level is abysmally low. Infrastructure presently available is not optimally utilized even in R&D systems.

Standards for information representation, sharing and management have not been evolved in spite of many projects. Reforms of administrative processes, control and human resources development are also the need of the hour. Gaps, deficiencies and barriers exist in the flow, dissemination and accessibility of fisheries information. Information services, skills to participate in the global information services, etc. are lacking in the sector. In India, there is no single point from which stakeholders can gather fisheries and farming related information. There is no information gateway service in the sector. Web-based advisory services especially for small-scale fisheries and aquaculture are almost absent in the sector. In Kerala, limited services are offered as a sub-set of *KissanKerala*. Nevertheless, the sector could not utilize the potential of *KissanKerala* or emulate it for other regions.

'Right to Information' is one of the driving forces for individual and societal development in a democratic nation. 'Fisheries Information' is the right of the stakeholders in the sector. Therefore, harnessing information with relevant technologies, services that are appropriate, business models that are scalable and regulatory environments that are applicable are to be ensured in the sector for information availability. Fisheries information sector is the least developed in whole of agricultural information systems. It is scattered between various government agencies, scientific and academic institutions and industry. Access to information depends upon the person's experience and their influences in the sector. Lack of information about socio-economic and cultural aspects of small-scale fisher communities obstruct decision and policy making. Language remains a challenge in flow of information. Information services in regional languages are very few. Multi language and translation services are absent in spite of technological, communication and software supports available.

Fisheries science being a specialized branch, networking of the institutions involved in R&D, Education and Training in the related areas is essential for fisheries development in the country. Information demand ranges from research to trade, from subjects as diverse as biology, economics, nutrition, environmental science, and social and cultural realms. The system resources, services, architecture and tools need to be strengthened, standardized, integrated and designed for use of primary stakeholders, administrators, scientists, teachers, students and marketing people with right combination of user needs, contents, hardware, software, cooperation of participating institutions and support of controlling/implementing agencies. By implementing an effective information system, the wide range of issues prevailing in fisheries information sector shall get addressed.

Stakeholders

The information resources are the stock-in-trade of state-funded libraries, research institutions and education institutions. The huge cost invested in these institutions is justified when the fruits of the institutional activities reach the stakeholders. There are no effective measures of reach of information resourced in these institutions to the grassroots and stakeholders. Fishers and fish farmers have a very few options for information access. The role of the village libraries in providing physical access to information are neglected by the local administration and primary societies. Physical access to information such as print pamphlets, radio broadcasts, rural libraries, etc. are important in the digital age also and are to be augmented. Low education levels of primary stakeholders, lack of delivery mechanisms, inadequate need assessment, etc. are the barriers in information dissemination to the primary stakeholders. Libraries and information centres of the national institutions and universities do not meet the information requirements of the primary stakeholders in reciprocation to the information resources built on public funds. According to the CGIAR Report, of the expected users of agriculture information systems, less than 1% constitutes scientists/administrators and 99% are farmers. (CGIAR 1989) Presently, information access is the privilege of the scientists who may or may not use it for the benefit of the farmers. Farmers need information for their entrepreneurial and livelihood issues but are not easy obtaining.

Libraries and Information Resource Sharing Networks

Awareness programmes are absent in the sectoral libraries. International resource sharing and information finding tools such as Directory of Open Access Journals (DOAJ), Journal Store (JSTOR), Google Scholar, International Network for the Availability of Scientific Publications (INASP); global information sources such as Network of Aquaculture Centre in Asia Pacific (NACA), Aquaculture Network Information Centre (AquaNIC), Centre for Environment, Fisheries and Aquaculture (CEFAS), CNREP, Centre for Maritime Research (MARE), Coral Reef Targeted Research and Capacity Building for Management (CRTR), Danish Institute of Fisheries Research (DIFR), EUROPA, FishBase, Fishermen and Scientists Research Society (FSRS), ICSF, ICES, International Institute of Fisheries Economics and Trade (IIFET), Indian Ocean and South-East Asian (IOSEA) Marine Turtle Memorandum of Understanding, World Aquaculture Society (WAS), etc., are not being reached to the information seekers. Informatics led services managed by libraries and information centres in the sector are very few. Participation in the global information resource sharing is weak in the sector. Institutional membership in IAMSLIC, Aquatic Commons, JSTOR, etc. is not common.

Library networks offer efficient and cost-effective means to share information. Therefore, library networks in the sector need strengthening with resources, professionalism, expertise and electronic connectivity. Food and livelihood security issues and the lack of extension support for fishers and fish farmers should be made up through information networks by combining mobile, cloud computing and newer networking technologies.

Orientation on resources, Portals, Open Access ETDs, Digital Archives, online services, etc. is not common in the sector. Training on access to discovery tools, bibliographic databases, web portals, information harvesters and search engines for finding relevant, timely and authoritative information efficiently and cost-effectively are not offered in the sector. Large number of Open Access sources in social, economic and management sciences are not brought to the notice of potential users. Stakeholders in the sector need skill development for accessing information effectively and efficiently.

Institutional libraries form the heart and lifeblood of information systems and are the agencies to manage information in the right way. Often, the library services are neglected in agricultural research system under ICAR, DAHDF and MoA. Libraries under these agencies are passive providers of routine services. Information resources and services that are to be integrated and harmonized with library and information systems are often kept separate like extension information, research information, etc. making them inaccessible to the stakeholders through the common information outlets. Libraries and information centres need to develop into a system for information management. The phenomenal development in computer and communication technology makes it possible to harmonize, integrate, disseminate and share information efficiently and effectively. Intangibles such as information, content creation, information transfer, standards, protocols etc are to be given more importance rather than tangibles in an information system lest it may fail to deliver information.

Agenda for National Fisheries Information Infrastructure

Development earmarked for fisheries sector need a strong backing of information and knowledge system. Flow of information in all directions need to be built to help the community of fishers and farmers for providing long-term gains. Welfare programmes have to be reoriented to provide empowerment of fishers and women in fisheries sector who remain poorest of poor and occupy lower status in the social strata. Weather forecast, fishery forecast, market intelligence, sustainable aquaculture, fish farming practices, disease diagnosis, health management, etc. need to reach the fish farmers and fishers well in time for long-term viability of fish farming, fishing and related operations. Portals are to be created for dissemination of information on these aspects so that fishers and fish farmers can access information directly or through NGOs, VKCs, VICs, extension workers, Department officers, etc.

The legal framework for the generation, distribution and use of fisheries information defined by various legislations are not comprehensive. Therefore, the National Fisheries Information Policy needs to be formulated. Its implementation shall enhance capabilities of the fisheries information system network and KGEU in fisheries sector. There is need to have effective mechanism to disseminate information to the primary audience and alternative audience especially of research output, laws and regulations relating to conservation and management operations. Flow of information which is almost linear in the sector should be made open and multi-directional so that flow of information between policy-makers, scientists, extension activists, fishing communities and other stakeholders is ensured. Open Access should be the guiding philosophy considering 'public good' nature of fisheries information. Digital services such as repositories, ETDs, archives and Open Access Journals are to be implemented in the sector.

Open Source web-enabled library management software should be developed by customizing from the existing ones or developing a new one for fisheries institutions. The software should support multiple Indian language scripts and full text linking. The software should facilitate networking and cloud computing. Potentials of cyber extension systems should be adopted in fisheries sector. Expertise gained in developing information exchange programmes such as *e-Krishi* and *Kissan Kerala* in the agricultural sector and such initiatives elsewhere needs to be adopted in fisheries sector. ETD of Mahatma Gandhi University, PFZ service of INCOIS, etc. are some of the models of digital information services for emulation. The Mobile telephony based services are also need to be introduced in fisheries sector.

Delivery of information in appropriate formats and languages needs to be ensured by the information systems and services in the sector. Immediate attention is needed in (i) providing context specific information; (ii) identifying and filling information gaps; (iii) enhancing access to information; (iv) using appropriate formats and dissemination methods and (v) ensuring multidirectional flow of information in order to meet the information requirements of the stakeholders including small-scale fisheries.

In order to increase openness and enhance accessibility, a series of web portals are to be created to aggregate, organize and present relevant and useful content in local languages in a uniform, customizable, user-friendly and personalized way. The portals have to serve as a single point of access for consolidated information, applications and resources of the sector. Computer facilities in the village schools could be modified to function as VKC/VIC/Internet access points at the grass-root levels. These centres should additionally provide a host of services on rural livelihood through access to information on finance, markets, insurance, healthcare and education to ensure regular usage by the primary stakeholders in the village.

Information services by harnessing latest technologies are to be planned and implemented in the sector. Mobile technology for delivering various government services through the Mobile Services Delivery Gateway (MSDG) should be extended to fishing villages. Value-added services by information providers and authentic services based on ***Aadhar*** are to be introduced. The service points for e-Governance in the Indian States (*Akshaya* centres in the State of Kerala) could also be modified to function as VKC/VIC in fishing villages. The potential of handheld devices such as mobile phone should be utilized to establish linkages and to share information and ideas among the stakeholders and change agents.

Libraries of the National fisheries institutions need to be heightened as Library and Information Divisions by building infrastructure, resources and networking. Human resources in fisheries libraries are to be revamped by revising the qualifications, methods for appointment, service conditions, etc. at par with scientists and academicians. Staffing, job descriptions, designations, pay scale, career advancement and service conditions of LIS Professionals in fisheries institutions should be re-assessed and revamped. CIFE library should be managed and administered as a University library.

Libraries need to be trained to make them relevant to user communities including fish farmers and fishers. It is observed that the controlling agencies pay scant regard for various reports of national standing like Report of the National Knowledge Commission, etc. The DAHDF should strengthen the libraries of institutions under them. ICAR, SAUs, CSIR and DST engaged in fisheries and allied research are to build strong cross-institutional interaction. The growing complexity of the information required for management and the high demand for information at national, regional and global level imply the development of collaborative information systems through which partners can join forces to produce comprehensive and integrated information resources. A high level committee under the Ministry of Agriculture should formulate norms and guidelines on working of the fisheries libraries on scientific lines. Management techniques such as brain storming and Delphi may be carried out for the purpose.

Interlibrary lending and cooperative development of library collections need to be promoted in the sector. It is feasible for a variety of cooperative endeavors to grow in ICT age. Willingness, the economic imperatives, formal and informal agreements, etc. are the pre-cursors for such initiatives. The major libraries in the sub-regions of India are to be made open to all in the sector and networked to the minor libraries in the region, so as to converge the minor libraries as information service outlets for better utilization of resources built up by public funds. Process of digitization also needs to be accelerated for resource sharing in a digital way, especially for documents generated in the different regions of India. Sensitization of user community on web based information services are also to be initiated in the sector.

National standards for interoperability of information resources and systems in fisheries informatics should be formulated to facilitate messaging, collation and analysis of data. The library operations and functions are to be standardized to provide effective library and information services. Norms and standards for document collection, staff, library budget, library services, etc. should be formulated and followed.

Adoption of international standards in the system smoothen the process of information exchange and pooling at institutional, State, national, regional and international levels. Therefore, mature standards such as NISO Z39.2 (MARC21) (for bibliographic information), Anglo-American Cataloguing Rules Second Edition (AACR-2) (for cataloguing), Commonwealth Agricultural Bureaux (CAB) Thesaurus (for subject descriptors), Z39.50 protocol (for remote bibliographic databases), Dublin Core (Z39.85) (to help catalog Internet resources), Open URL (Z39.88) (for encoding e-resource metadata within a URL), Open Archives Initiative Protocol for Metadata Harvesting (OAI-PMH) (for harvesting metadata from digital repositories), Common Communication Format, Common Command Language, and Unicode should be adopted for management of digital information. The system should also incorporate the newer ones at appropriate time. National Fisheries Information Policy should address these aspects, helping to evolve, transform and implement the National Fisheries Information Infrastructure.

Central Institution for Fisheries Informatics

There is an urgent need to build a Central institution focusing on fisheries informatics in order to ensure effective management of information in the sector. A robust, scientific and intensive Fisheries Information Network is indeed in need to promote transfer of information to all the stakeholders of the sector. There is also need to bring in economically viable fisher/farmer friendly models for efficient dissemination of fisheries related information including climate and weather risk warnings. An autonomous institution under DAHDF, MoA named as 'Central Institute of Fisheries Informatics' (CIFI) should be established for implementation of FISI. It will have the authority to ensure the smooth functioning of the Indian Fisheries Information System and Network named as 'Fisheries Information System Network' (FISNet). The institution so established shall deal with the problem of information dissemination in a more rational manner by streamlining the piecemeal and isolated activities performed now by different agencies. The CIFI should be the Centre of Excellence with high professional standing. Participation of a variety of people, including scientists, librarians, interface designers, ICT managers, software engineers, etc. should be ensured throughout design and development process of online tools and services of CIFI.

Central Institute of Fisheries Informatics should be established to deal with Fisheries Informatics with clear mandates and assigned responsibilities. CIFI should take leadership in designing and establishing the national fisheries information management system namely Fisheries Information System of India (FISI) which will be capable of organizing, harmonizing, integrating and disseminating all fisheries information in the country. CIFI's objectives should include in identifying critical issues needed in the design of the national fisheries information management system, identifying mechanisms for information gathering and disseminating within fisheries management information system, developing an integrated management information system and validating the system for fisheries sector. CIFI should act as a platform linking fisheries experts and field staff at various levels, State departments, District administration, SAUs, ICAR and other research institutions.

CIFI entrusted with the development and management of National Fisheries Portal should provide information contributed from different States and stakeholders on monthly, quarterly and annual basis. Research information and annual fisheries reports are also to be presented in suitable manner. It should implement modern mechanisms of disseminating analyzed information in the fisheries Management Information System and setting up central data bank that can be accessed online by Government stakeholders such as Departments at Centre and State, SAUs and other research and development institutions. CIFI should also function as National Repository of Bibliographic Records and the repository should contain records of bibliographic resources of fisheries science available in the country. Nodal centres should be responsible for creating bibliographic records. FISI shall function beyond dissemination of scientific information mode and transfer of technology mode so that the services shall also be relevant and useful to the primary stakeholders, helping them to make good decision through integration of different types of information served to them. Advanced Masters Degree courses on Fisheries Informatics should be offered by CIFI to meet the emerging requirements of professionals in the sector, to confront the developments in the informatics scenario in the world and to have a better system for fisheries information dissemination than what we have now. Academic Councils consisting of experts and academicians in the fields of LIS, ICT, Computer, Management and Fisheries should formulate course curriculum for fisheries informatics courses.

Areas of Further Research

Fisheries science is multi-disciplinary and it shares information and knowledge with numerous disciplines. Presently, the information services in different sub-systems of research, education, extension and socio-economic development work independently. They also duplicate resources and efforts at the cost of efficiency and effectiveness and causes waste of public funds. Therefore, harmonization and integration of fisheries information rest upon LIS professionals in the sector. Their efforts, in continuum, should be based on cooperation, resource sharing and modern ICT because fisheries information system is a neglected area of research. The institutional agencies for agriculture information - wherein fisheries is a sub set - generally neglect information professionals in the missions and programmes for information dissemination (ARIS of ICAR is an example). Managers often forget the extension workers, library and information resources, library services, LIS professionals, knowledge workers and primary stakeholders while implementing information networks and systems, due to lack of integrated view. These situations amply provide scope to the LIS Professionals for consortium based research in the areas of information science and fisheries information sector that shall contribute towards deliverance of efficient and effective information services. Earnest efforts in this direction can enable them to reinvent the professional concepts to demonstrate strategic and tactical value of the professional skill and they shall become the core part of Knowledge Management system in fisheries sector. In the immediate future, cloud computing that offers solutions in networking, cooperation, resource sharing and managing information resources is a virgin field for research.

Conclusion

The present study is an effort to map the status of information resources, services and systems in fisheries sector in India. It could identify the factors that hinder the nation for flow of information and from extracting optimum utility of the resources. The observations have helped in framing some of the fundamental solutions to improve the situation as well as for planning an integrated information system and resource sharing network for fisheries sector of the country. In order to accelerate the productivity and efficiency of fisheries research, education, extension and development, it is necessary to establish, develop and sustain an information system, specializing in fisheries. The study proposes Fisheries Information System by considering the fact that there is a serious constraint in the sector lacking systematic access to information. The problem is mainly with access to information rather than resources. The resources in the present form are also difficult for use by the stakeholders from the top to the grass root level as the sector lacks integration of information, information resource sharing, standards and protocols for information dissemination.

The practical value of the study, an academic exercise on the issues of fisheries information and knowledge systems, is for evolving policies to improve the system and services. The study puts forward some suggestions to the professionals, stakeholders concerned, administrators, and policy makers, who are earnestly working for establishing a Fisheries Information System. The noteworthy feature of the study is that it endorses and advocates for an equal opportunity for access to fisheries information to all concerned in the sector. The products generated by the study mainly include the schema of the proposed Fisheries Information System of India (FISI) besides recommendations for barrier free flow of fisheries information in the sector. The fisheries knowledge resources and information services aggregated during the study are given at Appendix 5 (International Institutions and Fisheries Information Web Resources) and Appendix 6 (Information System Services and Products for Finding Fisheries Information) The study explored aspects beyond the mere transactional and instrumental quality of the fisheries information sector to a more caring and humane system that enriches the lives of the fishers and fish farmers and make the social institutions responsible.

National agenda for revitalizing the library and information system in fisheries sector envisaged in this book is based on the detailed study of the present status of the system, technology and requirements. Implementation of these agendas can improve the quality, efficiency and cost effectiveness of library and information resources, services and system vis-à-vis sustainable development of the Indian fisheries sector. The knowledge managers and information service professionals have special responsibilities of collecting and conserving the knowledge resources on fisheries and in reaching the un-reached by offering very useful and important services to the fishing and fish farming communities. Providing information and knowledge of timely relevance to them can usher in a sense of credibility to the profession as well as transmit strength of knowledge to the communities for whom all these resources exist.

❑❑❑

References

Abdul Kalam, A.P.J. 2012. Empowering 3 Billion. *Address during valedictory session of 4th Organisation for Economic Co-operation and Development (OECD), 19 Oct 2012, New Delhi.* [Online]. Available at: http:// www.oecd.org/ site/worldforumindia/Adul%20 Kalam.pdf. [Accessed on 28 Dec 2012].

Abdul Kalam, A.P.J. 2011. Excerpts *Seafood News* 18-20 Feb 2011.

Agarwal, S.C. 2006. History of Indian Fishery, New Delhi: Daya Publishing.

AGMARKNET. 2013 [Online]. Available at: http://www.agmarknet.nic.in [Accessed on 23 Mar 2013]

Agropedia 2013 [Online]. Available at: http://agropedia.iitk.ac.in/. [Accessed on16 Feb 2013]

Anderson, Christa with Minasi, Mark. 1999. Local Area Networks. New York; Sybex Computer Books.

Anderson, Christopher M. 2011. Pathways to Better Outcomes for Fisheries. Conference on Fisheries Economics and Management-Future Challenges, 1-3 Sep 2011, Copenhagen. [Online]. Available at: http:// www. Foi.life.ku. dk/~/media/Foi/docs/ Aktiviteter/ Program_mv_Warming_2011.ashx. [Accessed on 23 Sep 2013].

Andrews, F.M., Klem, L., Davidson, T.N., O'Malley, P.M., and Rogers, W.L. 1981. A Guide for Selecting Statistical Techniques for Analysing Social Science Data., 2 ed. Ann Arbor, MI: Institute for Social Research, The University of Michigan.

Anjani Kumar et al. 2003. A Profile of People, Technologies and Policies in Fisheries Sector in India. New Delhi: National Centre for Agricultural Economics and Policy Research, p8.

Aruna, T.K and Pradhan S. 2006. Information and Communication Technology in Fisheries. In: Ayyappan et al. (Eds). *Handbook of*

Fisheries and Aquaculture. New Delhi: Indian Council of Agricultural Research, p 711-720.

Atherton, P. 1977. Handbook of Information Systems and Services. Paris: UNESCO.

Ayyappan, S and Diwan, A.D. 2007. National Fisheries Development Board and Fisheries Policy In: Vijayan, K.K. et al. (Eds). *Indian Fisheries-A Progressive Outlook*. Cochin: Central Marine Fisheries Research Institute.

Balaji, V. 2010. Director, Technology & Knowledge Management, Commonwealth of Learning, Vancouver, BC, Canada. *Interview* on 22 Nov 2010.

Bawden, David. 1990. User-oriented Evaluation of Information Systems and Services. Aldershot: Gower.

Bay of Bengal Programme -Inter-Governmental Programme. http://bobpigo.org/bobp-reports.html [Accessed on 11 Jan 2013].

Bernus, P., Mertins, K., and Schmidt, G. (Eds).2006. Handbook on Architectures of Information Systems, 2 ed. London: Springer.

Bhathal, B. 2004. Historical Reconstruction of Indian Marine Fisheries catches, 1950-2000, as basis for testing Marine Trophic Index. MSc thesis, Canada: University of British Columbia, p130.

Bhose, Joel S.G.R. 2003. NGOs and Rural Development: Theory and Practice. New Delhi: Concept Publication, p 18.

Bilio, M., Rosenthal, H and Sinderman, C.J. (Eds). 1981. Constaints, Perspectives. *Summary Statement, World Conference on Aquaculture, Venice, Italy, 21-25 September*. Rome: Food and Agriculture Organization, p 577-586.

Biotechnology Information System Network. http://www.btisnet.gov.in/ [Accessed on 23 Mar 2013]

Biradar, R.S. 2000. Fisheries Databases in India, *Indian Society of Fisheries Professionals Newsletter*, 2 (2), p17-18.

Biradar, R.S. 2006. Fisheries Education in India. In: Ayyappan, S et al, (Ed). *Handbook of Fisheries and Aquaculture*. New Delhi: Indian Council of Agricultural Research, p 659.

BOBP. 1992. Report of the Sixteenth Meeting of the Advisory Committee Jan 20-23, 1992, Phuket, Thailand. Madras: Bay of Bengal Programme.

Bodiguel, C. et al 2009. Actors of Un-sustainability and Overexploitation in Marine Fisheries, Rome: Food and Agriculture Organization.

Bogdan, R. and Taylor, S. 1975. Introduction to Qualitative Research Method. New York: John Wiley and Sons.

Busha, C.H. 1980. Research Methods in Librarianship: Techniques and Interpretation. London: Academic Press Inc.

Business Directory. 2011 [Online]. Available at: http://www. Businessdictionary. Com/definition/ information.html. [Accessed on 20 Sep 2010].

CABI. 2013 [Online]. Available at: http://www.cabi.org/services/knowledge-management-services/mobile-advisory-services/ [Accessed on 22 Mar 2013]

CARI 2007 Annual Report 2005-06.Port Blair; Central Agricultural Research Institute. p 70-78.

CARI 2011. Annual Report 2010-11. Port Blair: Central Agricultural Research Institute.

Carole, R, Engle and Nathan, M Stone. 1989. A Review of Extension Methodologies in Aquaculture. Rome: Food and Agriculture Organization.

CEL KAU 2013 [Online]. Available at http://www.celkau.in/ [Accessed on 14 Feb 2013]

Central Food Technological Research Institute http://www.cftri.res.in. [Accessed on 09 Nov 2012].

Central Institute of Coastal Engineering for Fishery. http://www.cicef.gov.in. [Accessed on 21 Sep 2012].

Centre for Development Studies http://www.cds.edu/. [Accessed on 14 Feb 2013].

Centre for Fisheries Studies http://www.cfs.archtvm.in. [Accessed on 02 Feb 2013].

Centre for Marine Living Resources and Ecology. http://cmlre.gov.in. [Accessed on 18 May 2012].

CeRA.2013 [Online]. Available at: http://cera.iari.res.in/attachments/article/19/cera%20leaflet-2012-FINAL.pdf [Accessed on22 Mar 2013]

CGIAR. 1989. Report of Consultative Group on International Agricultural Research on Agricultural Research Information System for India. New Delhi; Government of India.

Chitranshi, V.R. 2006. Oxbow Lake Fisheries. In: Ayyappan, S et al (Ed). *Handbook of Fisheries and Aquaculture*. New Delhi: Indian Council of Agricultural Research, p196-207.

Choudhury, S. et al. 2007. Validation of Integrated Potential Fishing Zone (IPFZ) Forecast using Satellite based Chlorophyll and Sea Surface Temperature along the East Coast of India. *International Journal of Remote Sensing* 28(12), p 2683-2693.

Churchman, C. West. 1968. The Systems Approach. New York: Delacorte Press. p.29.

CIBA. 2012. Annual Report 2011-12. Chennai: Central Institute of Brackishwater Aquaculture.

CIBRC. 2013 [Online]. Available at: http://cibrc.nic.in [Accessed on24 Mar 2013]

CIFA. 2012. Annual Report 2011-12. Bhubaneswar: Central Institute of Freshwater Aquaculture.

CIFE. 2012. Annual Report 2011-12. Versova: Central Institute of Fisheries Education.

CIFNET. 2011. Annual Report 2010-11. Cochin: Central Institute of Fisheries Nautical and Engineering Training.

CIFRI. 2012. Annual Report 2011-12. Barrackpore: Central Inland Capture Fisheries Research Institute.

CIFT. 2012. Annual Report 2011-12. Cochin: Central Institute of Fisheries Technology.

Clarke, K.C. 1986. Recent Trends in Geographic Information System Research, *Geoprocessing* 3, p1-15.

Cleland, D.I. and King, W.R. 1969. Systems, Organizations, Analysis and Management:A Book of Reading. New York: McGraw Hill Book Company. p64.

CMFRI. 2012A. Annual Report 2011-12. Cochin: Central Marine Fisheries Research Institute.

CMFRI. 2012B. Mandapam Regional Centre Library Goes Online. *CMFRI Newsletter No. 135*, Oct-Dec 2012. Cochin: Central Marine Fisheries Research Institute, p15.

Coastal Aquaculture Authority http://www.caa.gov.in [Accessed on 28 Jun 2013]

Cochrane, L Kevern and Garcia, Serge Michel. 2009. Fisheries Management. In: Cochrane, K. L. and Garcia, S.M.(Ed). *A Fishery Manager's Guidebook*, 2nd ed, Rome: Food and Agriculture Organization and Wiley-Blackwell.

Coordinator Kissan Kerala. 2011. *Brochure.* Thiruvananthapuram: Kissan Operations Centre.

Crag, Robert T. 1999. Communication Theory as a Field. *Communication Theory* 9(2), p 161-199.

CUSAT. 2007. *Brochure*, Cochin: Faculty of Marine Sciences, Cochin University of Science and Technology. pp 5.

DACNET. 2013 [Online]. Available at: http://dacnet.nic.in [Accessed on 23 Mar 2013].

DAHDF. 2009. Handbook on Fisheries Statistics 2008. New Delhi: Department of Animal Husbandry, Dairying and Fisheries, Government of India, p 5-97.

Day, Francis. 1883. The Fishes of India; being a Natural History of the Fishes known to inhabit the Seas and Fresh Waters of India, Burma and Ceylon. Reprint 1978. New Delhi: Today and Tomorrow's Book Agency.

DCFR. 2012. Annual Report 2011-12. Bhimtal: Directorate of Coldwater Fisheries Research.

Dehadrai, P.V. 2005. Women at the Centre Stage for Socio-Economic Change in Fishing Community. In: Ninawe, A.S. and Diwan, A.D. (Eds). *Women Empowerment in Fisheries*. New Delhi: Narendra Publishing.

Dehadrai, P.V. 2006. Indian Fisheries Resources and Production. In: Ayyappan, S et al. (Eds). *Handbook of Fisheries and Aquaculture*. New Delhi: Indian Council of Agricultural Research, p. 1-30.

Desai, V.R. 2006. Reservoir Fisheries. In: Ayyappan, S et al. (Eds). *Handbook of Fisheries and Aquaculture.* New Delhi: Indian Council of Agricultural Research, p 173-195.

Deshmukh, P.P. 1990. Standardization of Library and Information Services with Special Reference to Science and Agriculture Libraries. New Delhi: ABC Publications. p57.

Devarajan, G and Joseph Kurien, P. 2011. Information Access, Tools, Services and Systems. New Delhi: EssEss Publications. p. 197.

Devarajan, G. 2000. Information Technology for Agricultural Development. In: *Agricultural Information Systems: Vision 2020*, Thrissur: IASLIC Study Circle, p6.

Devarajan, G. 2011. Prolegomena to Research Methodology. New Delhi; Ess Ess Publications.

Dillman, D.A. 1978. The Mail and Telephone Survey: The Total Design Method. New York: Wiley-Interscience.

DPPQS. 2013 [Online]. Available at: http://ppqs.gov.in [Accessed on 24 Mar 2013].

Duran, C. 1991. The Role of LIS Education. In: McClure, C.R. and Hernon, P. (Eds). *Library and Information Science Research: Perspective and Strategies for Improvement*. Norwood: Ablex Publishing, p. 147-159.

Export Inspection Council of India. http://www.eicindia.gov.in. [Accessed on 13 Feb 2013].

FAO. 1976. Report of the FAO Technical Conference on Aquaculture, Kyoto, Japan, 28 May-2 Jun 1976. *Fish Report 188*. Rome: Food and Agriculture Organization.

FAO. 1995. Code of Conduct for Responsible Fisheries. Rome: Food and Agriculture Organization, Fisheries and Aquaculture Department [Online]. Available at: http://www.fao.org/fishery/code/en. [Accessed on 28 Dec 2012].

FAO. 2001. Fisheries and Aquaculture Topics: Fisheries Governance [Online]. Available at: http://www.fao.org/fishery/topic/2014/en. [Accessed on 25 Aug 2012].

FAO. 2002. Fisheries Statistics and Information. Rome: FAO Fisheries and Aquaculture Department [Online]. Available at: http:/ www. Fao. Org/fishery/topic/2017/en. [Accessed on 25 Aug 2012].

FAO. 2004. Report of and Papers Presented at the Regional Workshop on Networking for Improved Access to Fisheries and Aquaculture Information in Africa. FAO Fisheries Report No.740. Rome: Food and Agriculture Organization.

FAO. 2005. Fisheries and Aquaculture Topics: Future Challenges for the CWP [Online]. Available at: http://www.fao.org/fishery/cwp/future-challenges/en. [Accessed on 28 Dec 2012]

FAO. 2009. Information and Knowledge Sharing, FAO Fisheries Technical Guidelines for Responsible Fisheries No. 12. Rome: Food and Agriculture Organization.

FAO. 2011. Information and Communications Technologies (ICT) in Institutional Websites. [Online]. Available at: http://www.fao.org/fishery/topic/16618/en. [Accessed on 28 Dec 2011].

FAO. 2012. [Online]. Available at: http: //www.fao.org/docrep/003/W4493E/w4493e03.htm [Accessed on 28 Dec 2012].

FAO. 2013. [Online]. Available at: http://www.fao.org/fishery/topic/16073 [Accessed on 23 Mar 2013].

FishBase. 2011. [Online]. Available at: http://www.fishbase.org. [Accessed on 20 Sep 2011].

FSI. 2006. Profile 1946-2006. *Brochure*. Mumbai: Fishery Survey of India.

FSI. 2011. Annual Report 2010-11. Mumbai: Fishery Survey of India.

Geoffery J.M and Thang D.C. 1996. Geographical Information Systems – Applications to Marine Fisheries. *FAO Fisheries Technical Paper T 356*. Rome: FAO, pp 335.

Ghosh, B.N. 1982. Scientific Methods and Social Research. New Delhi: Sterling Publishers.

Government of India. 1976. Report of the National Commission on Agriculture-Part VIII, Fisheries. New Delhi: Ministry of Agriculture.

Government of India. 2008. Handbook on Fisheries Statistics. New Delhi: DAHDF.

Government of India. 2010. Statistical System in India: 2009. New Delhi: Ministry of Statistics and Programme Implementation. p 191.

Government of India. 2012. Fisheries [Online]. Available at: http://india.gov.in/sectors/agriculture/fisheries.php. [Accessed on 12 Apr 2012].

Government of India. 2012A. Annual Report 2011-12 Department of Animal Husbandry, Dairying and Fisheries. New Delhi: Ministry of Agriculture, p 51.

Government of India. 2012B. Economic Survey 2010-11. New Delhi: Ministry of Agriculture.

Government of India. 2013 [Online]. Available at: http://india.gov.in. [Accessed on 04 Jan 2013]

Government of Kerala, 1969. Master Plan for Fisheries Development-Kerala State. Trivandrum: Directorate of Fisheries.

Government of Kerala. 2009. Kerala Inland Fisheries Statistics. Thiruvananthapuram: Department of Fisheries.

Government of Kerala. 2010A. Kerala Marine Fisheries Statistics. Thiruvananthapuram: Department of Fisheries.

Government of Kerala. 2010B. Government Farms and Hatcheries of Kerala. Thiruvananthapuram: Department of Fisheries.

Government of Kerala. 2011. [Online]. Available at: http://www. fisheries. kerala. gov.in/[Accessed on 30 Dec 2011].

Government of Kerala. 2012. [Online]. Available at:http:// www.kerala.gov.in/index.php?option=com_content. [Accessed on 10 Dec 2012].

Government of Kerala. 2013. [Online]. Available at http://www. old.kerala.gov.in/dept_fisheries.htm. [Accessed on 18 Feb 2013].

Gupta, T.R.C. 2006. Estuarine Fisheries. In: Ayyappan, S et al. (Eds). *Handbook of Fisheries and Aquaculture*. New Delhi: Indian Council of Agricultural Research. p 158-172.

Hasan, Nabi. 2012. Web-based Agricultural Information Systems and Services under National Agricultural Research System. *DESIDOC Journal of Library & Information technology*, 32(1), p 24-30.

Hirwade, Mangala and Hirwade, Anil. 2012. Traditional Knowledge Protection: An Indian Prospective. *DESIDOC Journal of Library & Information Technology*, 32(3), p 240-248.

Hora, S.L. 1948. Knowledge of the Ancient Hindus concerning fish and fisheries of India reference to fish in Arthasastra (Ca 300B.C.). Kolkata: *JAS Bengal (letters)*, 1(1), p 7-10.

Horton, F. W. Jr. 1974. How to Harness Information Resources: A Systems Approach. Cleveland, Ohio: Association for Systems Management.

IAMSLIC. 2013 [Online]. Available at http: //www. iamslic. org. [Accessed on 24 Mar 2013].

Ibeun, M.O. 2004. Information Needs and Feasibility for a National Focal Point for the Exchange of Inland Fisheries and Aquaculture Information in Nigeria, FAO Fisheries Report No. 740. Rome: Food and Agriculture Organization, p 81-97.

ICAR *e-Granth*. 2013 [Online]. Available at: http://egranth.ac.in/ ?q=AboutUs. [Accessed on 20 Mar 2013].

ICAR. 1975. Report of the Regional Agricultural Study and Survey Team. New Delhi: Indian Council of Agricultural Research.

ICAR. 2010. ICT/ICM Initiatives for Agricultural R&D. *ICAR News*. Jul-Sep 2010. New Delhi: Indian Council of Agricultural Research.

ICAR. 2012. ICAR Fisheries Division at a Glance. *Brochure*. New Delhi: Indian Council of Agricultural Research.

ICAR. 2013.[Online]. Available at: http://www.icar.org.in/node/1238. [Accessed on 23 Mar 2013].

ICSF. 2011. Indian Fisheries [Online]. Available at: http://indianfisheries.icsf.net/ en/page/614-Fisheries% 20 Development% 20and%20 Management.html [Accessed on 28 Jul 2011].

ICSF. 2013. [Online]. Available at: http://indianfisheries.icsf.net/en/page/827-Indian%20Legal%20Instruments.html. [Accessed on 28 Feb 2013].

INCOIS. 2007. Potential Fishing Zone Advisory Services. *Ocean News*. 1(1), p 2.

Indian Agricultural Research Institute http://www.iari.res.in [Accessed on 29 Dec 2012].

Indian Agricultural Statistics Research Institute. http://www.iasri.res.in. [Accessed on 12 Oct 2011].

Indian Council for Agricultural Research. http:// www.icar.org. [Accessed on 29 Dec 2011].

Indian Institute of Foreign Trade. http://www.iift.edu. [Accessed on 24 Feb 2013].

Indian Institute of Management Ahemedabad. 1984. Marine Fish Marketing in India. Vol 1-6. New Delhi: Concept Publishing.

Indian Institute of Management Ahemedabad. 1985. Inland Fish Marketing in India. Vol 1-8 New Delhi: Concept Publishing.

Indian Institute of Packaging. http://www.iip-in.com/ [Accessed on 24 Feb 2013].

Indian National Centre for Ocean Information System. http://www.incois.gov.in/Incois/marine_fisheries_main.jsp [Accessed on 24 Mar 2013].

Indo-American Agricultural Library Survey and Study Team. 1969. Final Report on the ICAR Institutes and Agricultural University Libraries. New Delhi: Indian Council of Agricultural Research.

Jayakrishnan, J. S. 2013. Kerala Public Library Network: A Project Report [Online] Available at eprints.rclis.org/20451/1/KPLNET.pdf. [Accessed on 30 Sep 2013].

Jayapradeep, M and Raman Nair, R. 2012A. Survey of Aquatic and Fisheries Information System Capacity in the Region of Cochin, Kerala. *SRELS Journal of Information Management*, 49(5), p 511-527.

Jayapradeep, M and Raman Nair, R. 2012B. Need for Knowledge Management in Fisheries Sector: An area of Cooperation among SAARC Countries. In: Rishi Tiwari et al (Eds). *Trends and Development in Library and Information Science: Proceedings of the SAARC Conference for Library and Information Professionals, Dec 01-02, 2012*. New Delhi: Zenith Publications.

Jayasree, B and Subbia, A. 2000. Mapping Fish Research in India. *Current Science*. 79(5), p 613-620.

Jha, Ashok Kumar. 2004. Sustainable Development: Concept and Strategies. Delhi: Adhyayan Publications.

Jhingran, V.G. 1975. Fish and Fisheries of India. Delhi: Hindustan Publishing Corporation.

Johannes, R.E. 2003. Fishers Knowledge and Management: Differing Fundamentals in Artisanal and Industrial Fisheries In: *Fisheries Center Research Reports 11 (1) :15-19*. Vancouver BC: University of British Columbia Press.

Johnson, E. 1986. Design and Development of National Information System for Marine Fisheries in India. Ph D Thesis. Trivandrum: University of Kerala.

Joice, V.T., Deepu A.V. and Afsal, V.V. 2010. Annual Report 2008-09: Network for Fish Quality Management and Sustainable Fishing. Ernakulam: Marine Products Export Development Authority, p 4-5.

Kadzamira, G.A., Ngwira, M.E. and Salanje, G.F. 2004. Review of the Fisheries Information Resources in Malawi: Case study. FAO Fisheries Report No. 740. Rome: Food and Agriculture Organization, p 61-80.

Kapoor, D., Dayal, R. and Ponniah, A.G. 2002. Fish biodiversity of India. Lucknow: National Bureau of Fish Genetic Resources, p 75.

KAU. 2008. Annual Report 2007-08. Thrissur, Kerala Agricultural University.

Kelly, R.J. Keynote Address by the Minister for the Arts, Sport and the Environment and Territories. 1992. *The Earth Summit, the UN Conference on the Environment and Development(UNCED) Rio de Janeiro, Brazil Jun 3-14, Canberra.* Geneva: UNO.

Kerala Agricultural University. http://www.kau.edu. [Accessed on 22 Jan 2013].

Kerala Forest Research Institute. http://www.kfri.org/. [Accessed on 25 Jan 2013].

Kerala Institute for Entrepreneurship Development. http://www.kied.info. [Accessed on 25 Jan 2013].

Kerala Rural Employment and Welfare Society. http://www.krews.co.in. [Accessed on 25 Jan 2013].

Kerala State Cooperative Federation for Fisheries Development Limited. http://www.matysafed.org. [Accessed on 12 Feb 2013].

Kerala State Planning Board. 2006. Human Development Report 2005 Prepared by Centre for Development Studies. Trivandrum: Government of Kerala.

KIED. 2007. Kerala Fisheries. Thiruvananthapuram, Kerala Institute for Environment and Development.

Kissan Kerala. 2013. [Online]. Available at: http://www.kissankerala.net/ . [Accessed: 28 Jan 2013].

Kochtanek, Thomas R and Matthews, Joseph R. 2002. Library Information Systems: From Library Automation to Distributed Information Access Solutions. Connecticut: Libraries Unlimited.

Koontz, H and Weihrich, H. 1990. Essentials of Management, 5 ed. Singapore: McGraw-Hill Book Co.

Korakandy, Ramakrishnan. 1994. Technological Change and the Development of Marine Fishing Industry in India. New Delhi: Daya Publishing, p 19.

Kothari, C.R. 2004. Research Methodology: Methods and Techniques., 2 ed. New Delhi: New Age International Publishers.

Krishan Kumar. 1992. Research Methods in Library and Information Science. New Delhi: Har- Anand Publications.

Krishnaiah, P. 2010. Interview with NFDB Chief Executive. *The Practical Asian Aquaculture.* 1(2).

KUFOS. 2011. Academic Brochure 2011-12. Kochi, Kerala University of Fisheries and Ocean Studies.

Lancaster, F. W. 1977. The Measurement and Evaluation of Library Services. Washington: Information Resources Press.

Library. Indian Agricultural Science and Research Institute. http://lib.iasri.res.in/*krishiprabha*.asp [Accessed on 21 Mar 2013].

M S Swaminathan Research Foundation. http://www.mssrf.org/. [Accessed on 26 Nov 2012].

Malabar Coastal Institute for Training, Research and Action. http://www.mcitra.org. [Accessed on 27 Jan 2013].

Malhotra, S.P and Sinha, V.R.P. 2007. Indian Fisheries and Aquaculture in a Globalising Economy. New Delhi: Narendra Publications.

Mangala, P.B. 2003. Information Society, Information Systems and National Development: A Conceptual Approach. *Annals of Library and Information Science*, 53 (2), p 56-58.

Mann, E. J. 2014. Focus on Agricultural Information Transfer. *Informatics Studies* 1(1), p 50-55.

Mashelkar, R.A. 1999. Economics of Knowledge. *Current Science*. 77(2), p 228.

Mauch, James E and Birch, Jack W. 1998. Guide to the Successful Thesis and Dissertation: A Handbook for Students and Faculty, 4 e. New York. Marcel Dekker.

Maunder, A.H. 1973. Agricultural Extension: A Reference Manual (abridged edition). Rome: Food and Agriculture Organization.

McConney, Patrick and Haynes, Carmel. 2011. Communication. In: Pomeroy, Robert S and Andrew, Neil. (Eds). *Small-scale Fisheries Management: Frameworks and Approaches for the Developing World*. Oxfordshire: CAB International, p 178-195.

Meloy, J. 1994. Writing the Qualitative Dissertation. Mahwah, NJ: Lawrence Erlbaum Associates, Inc.

Metkewar, P.S. and Acharya, H.S. 2006. Agro Information System: Identification and Parameterization of Needs of Farmers, Planners and Research Workers. Lucknow: IBDC Publication.

Miller, D.C. 1985. Handbook of Research Design and Social Measurement., 4 ed. New York: McKay.

Mingers, John and Stowell, Frank. 1997. Information Systems: An emerging discipline?.London; McGraw-Hill.

Mishra, B. K. 2011. Managing Director, FISHCOPFED. *Interview* on 10 Sep 2011.

MoES. 2013 [Online]. Available at: http://moeseprints.incois.gov.in/information.htm [Accessed on 24 Mar 2013].

Moni, M. 2004. Agricultural Informatics and Communication Network (AGRISNET): An ICT Infrastructure to usher in Digital Opportunities for Sustainable Agricultural Development in India. In: Sundaram, K.V., Moni, M and Jha, M., (Eds). *Natural Resources Management and Livelihood Security: Survival Strategies and Sustainable Policies.* New Delhi: Concept Publishing, p 378-397.

MPEDA. 2009. Export Trend of Marine Products. Cochin: Marine Products Export Development Authority.

MPEDA. 2012. Annual Report 2011-12. Cochin: Marine Products Export Development Authority.

MSSRF, 2001. Chennai Declaration. *MSSRF-FAO Expert Consultation on Science for Sustainable Food Security, Nutritional Adequacy and Poverty Alleviation in the Asia-Pacific Region, 25-28 Jun 2001.* Chennai: MS Swaminathan Research Foundation.

NAARM. 2012. Annual Report of the National Academy of Agricultural Research Management for 2011-12. Hyderabad: National Academy of Agricultural Research Management.

National Centre for Earth Sciences Studies. http://cess.res.in. [Accessed on 20 Feb 2013].

National Commission on Agriculture. 1976. *Report : Part VIII- Fisheries.* New Delhi: Government of India, Ministry of Agriculture and Irrigation.

National Federation of Fishermen's Cooperatives Ltd. http://fishcopfed.com [Accessed on 25 May 2013]

National Information Centre for Marine Science. http://www.nio.org/nicmas [Accessed on 12 Dec 2012].

National Institute of Agricultural Extension Management. http://www.manage.gov.in. [Accessed on 20 Feb 2012].

National Institute of Nutrition. http://www.ninindia.org. [Accessed on 18 Sep 2012].

National Institute of Ocean Technology. http://www.niot.res.in. [Accessed on 17 Oct 2012].

National Institute of Oceanography. http://www.nio.org [Accessed on 23 Mar 2013].

National Institute of Rural Development and Panchayatiraj. http://www.nird.gov.in. [Accessed on 20 Feb 2012].

National Remote Sensing Agency. http://www.nrsa.gov.in. [Accessed on 12 Jan 2013].

NBFGR. 2011. Vision 2030. *Brochure*. Lucknow: National Bureau of Fish Genetic Resources.

NBFGR. 2012. Annual Report 2011-12. Lucknow: National Bureau of Fish Genetic Resources.

NCAER. 2010. Impact Assessment and Economic Benefits of Weather and Marine Services. New Delhi: National Council of Applied Economic Research, p 4.

NCAP. 2013. Annual Report 2011-12. New Delhi: National Centre for Agricultural Economics and Policy Research.

Nehru Library. 2014. [Online]. Available at: http: // 14. 139. 232. 167.: 8080/ HUA/thesis. html [Accessed on 10 Jan 2014]

Netfish. 2013. Annual Report 2011-12. Ernakulam: Network for Fish Quality Management and Sustainable Fishing.

NFDB. 2009. Indian Fisheries. *Brochure*. Hyderabad: National Fisheries Development Board.

NICMAS. 2013. [Online]. Available at: http://www.nio.org/index/option/com_nomenu/task/show/tid/1/sid/12/id/64 [Accessed on 24 Mar 2013].

NIFARM 2013. [Online]. Available at: http://www.fisheries.kerala.gov.in/ Index.php?options=com_content &view=article&id=114&Itemid=77. [Accessed on 18 Sep 2013].

NIFPHATT. 2011. Annual Report 2010-11. Cochin: National Institute of Fisheries Post Harvest Technology and Training.

NISO. 2013 [Online]. Available at http://www.niso.org/whatare.html [Accessed on 20 Jan 2013].

NKN. 2013 [Online]. Available at: http://www.nkn.in/ download.php?file=NKN_Brochure.pdf. [Accessed on 25 Mar 2013].

OCLC. 2012. [Online]. Available at: http:// www.oclc.org/worldcat/join/default.htm. [Accessed on 13 Apr 2012].

Olena Y, Korchaka. 2006. Encyclopaedia of Social Sciences: Economics. Delhi: IVY Publications.

Oommen, M.A. 1999. Kerala's Development Experience. New Delhi: Concept Publishing.

Panda, S.K. 2009. Capture Fishery Resources of India. In: Meenakumari et al. (Eds). *Handbook of Fishing Technology*. Cochin: Central Institute of Fisheries Technology.

Pillai, N.G.K and Katiha, P.K. 2004. Evolution of Fisheries and Aquaculture in India. Kochi: Central Marine Fisheries Research Institute.

Planning Commission. 2001. Report of the Working Group on Fisheries for the Tenth Five Year Plan: TFYP Working Group Sr. No. 16/ 2001. [Online]. Available at: http://planningcommission.gov.in/aboutus/committee/ wrkgrp/ fishery.pdf. [Accessed on 16 Jul 2012]

Planning Commission. 2010. Towards faster and more inclusive growth – An approach to the 11th Five Year Plan. New Delhi: Government of India.

Pomeroy, R.S. and Rivera-Guieb, R. 2005. Fishery co-management: A Practical Handbook. New York: CAB International.

Powell, Ronald R. 1985. Basic Research Methods for Librarians. New Jersey: Ablex Publishing.

Prytherch, Raymond John. 2005. Harrod's Librarians' Glossary and Reference Book : A Dictionary of over 10,200 terms, organizations, projects and acronyms in the areas of Information Management, Library Science, Publishing and Archive Management.,10th ed. Hampshire: Ashgate

Radack, Shirley M. 1990. More Effective Federal Computer Systems: The Role of NIST and Standards. *Government Information Quarterly*. 7(1), p. 38.

Raghu Prakash, R. 2009. Application of Geographic Information System in Fisheries Management. In: Meenakumari, B. et al.(Eds). *Handbook of Fishing Technology*. Cochin: Central Institute of Fisheries Technology, p 316-322.

Rajagopalan, T.S. and Rajan, T.N. 1986. National Information Policy for India: A Perspective. In: Gupta, B.M. (Ed). *Handbook of Libraries,*

Archives and Information Centres in India., Vol 3 Information Policy, Systems and Networks. New Delhi: Information Industry Publications, p 67.

Rajaraman, V. 2014. Cloud Computing. *Resonance,* 19(3), p 242-257.

Ralph, Shaw. R. and Krishna Rao, D.B. 1957. Report on Library and Bibliographical Services for Agricultural Teaching and Research in India. New Delhi: Indian Council of Agricultural Research.

Ramachandran, C. 2004. Teaching Not to F(in)ish: A Constructivist Perspective on Reinventing a Responsible Marine Fisheries Extension System. Kochi: Central Marine Fisheries Research Institute.

Ramakrishnan, K. 2010. Fisheries Development in India: The Political Economy of Unsustainable Development, 2 volumes. Delhi: Kalpaz Publications.

Raman Nair, R 2012. Information System Expert and Former University Librarian, Kerala Agricultural University. *Interview* on 24 Dec 2012.

Raman Nair, R. 2000. Who should Manage Information Technology Development. In: *Agricultural Information Systems: Vision 2020.* Thrissur: IASLIC Study Circle, p 7-15.

Raman Nair, R. 2004. An Investigative and Evaluative Study of Factors Affecting Quality of Agricultural and Farm Information Services in Kerala.*Ph D Thesis.* Trivandrum: University of Kerala.

Raman Nair, R. 2007. Information Resources and Services on Aqua Sciences and Fisheries in India. *Library Herald* 45(3), p 225-248.

Randhawa, M.S. 1986. A History of Agriculture in India, Vol. IV. New Delhi: Indian Council of Agricultural Research. p 606-610.

Ratzan, Lee. 2009. Understanding Information Systems. New Delhi: Indiana Publishing House, p 253.

Ravisankar, T., Rajukumar, S., and Shenbagakumar. M . 2004. Open Access and Information sharing for Responsible Aquaculture Development. In: *Information and Communication Technology for Agricultural and Rural Development.* Hyderabad: National Academy of Agricultural Research Management.

Rawat, P.P. and Kumar, T. 2002. Encyclopedic Dictionary of Library Science and Information Technology, New Delhi: Crest Publishing House, pp 1145.

ReALCraft 2013 [Online]. Available at: http://fishcraft.nic.in. [Accessed on 12 Sep 2013]

Regional Agricultural Research Station. Kerala Agricultural University http:// www.kau.edu/ rarskumarakom.htm. [Accessed on 21 Dec 2012].

Regional centre. Zoological Survey of India. http://www.zsi.gov.in/ regional_centres/ wgrc_calicut.html. [Accessed on 27 Jan 2013].

RGCA. 2013. [Online]. Available at: http://www.rgca.org.in/ institutional.php. [Accessed on 20 Apr 2013].

Rizvi, Haider S.M and Dearden, Andy. 2012. Knowledge Help Extension Technology Initiative (KHETI) - A Participatory Interactive ICT Designed Solution in Agriculture for Livelihoods Promotions. [Online] Available at: http://www.iimahd.ernet.in/egov/ifip/ oct2010/syed-rizvi.htm. [Accessed on 03 Apr 2013].

Royce, F William. 1984. Introduction to the Practice of Fishery Science. London: Academic Press.

Sahrhage, D. 1992. The Role of Science in International Management of Fish Resources. In: Andresen, S smf W Ostreng. (Ed). *International Resource Management: the Role of Science and Politics*. New Delhi: CBS Pubications.

Sanjeeva Ghosh, D. 2007. Data Needs and Gaps in Kerala Fisheries. In Ramachandran Nair, G and Rajan, J.B. (Eds). *Kerala Fisheries: Exploring Data Needs for Resource Management*. Thiruvananthapuram; Kerala Institute for Environment and Development, p 15-23.

Sankar Rao, D.V. and Raju, V.T. 1998. Economics of Fisheries Technologies. Jaipur: Ambika Book Agency.

Sardana, J.L. and Sehgal, R.L. 1982. Statistical Methods for Librarians. New Delhi: Ess Ess Publications.

Sarkar, S.K., De, H.K., Saha, G.S and Kuldeep Kumar. 2007. Fisheries Extension. In: Ayyappan et al, (Eds). *Handbook of Fisheries and Aquaculture*. New Delhi: Indian Council of Agricultural Research, pp 644.

Satija, M.P. 2003. Digital Information Systems and Services. *Library Times International*, 11(2), p 24-26.

Satyanarayana, R. 1993. Education for Information Resource Management. In: Karisiddappa, C.R., Sangam, S.L. and Maheswarappa, B.S. (Eds).

Current Studies in Library and Information Science. Delhi: Manak Publications, p 132.

Seafood Exporters Association of India http://seai.in. [Accessed on 15 Nov 2012].

Senthilkumaran, S. 2011. Village Knowledge Centres and Village Resource Centres- An Overview. In Saravanan, R., Kathiresan, C. and Indira Devi, T. (Eds). *Information and Communication Technology for Agriculture and Rural Development*. New Delhi; New India Publishing Agency, p 77-99.

Shakshuki, E., Ghenniwa, H. and Kamel, M. 2003. An Architecture for Cooperative Information Systems; *Knowledge Based Systems*, 3(2), p-12.

SICOM. 2010. Coastal Management. *Newsletter* 1(1) Oct 2010. New Delhi: Society of Integrated Coastal Management.

Silas, E.G. (Ed) 1977. Indian Fisheries 1947-77. Cochin: Central Marine Fisheries Research Institute.

Sinha, M. 2006. Riverine Fisheries of India. In: Ayyappan, S et al. (Eds). *Handbook of Fisheries and Aquaculture*. New Delhi: Indian Council of Agricultural Research, p 142-157.

Sinha, V.R.P. 2005. Fisheries Research Planning and Management in Developing Countries. New Delhi: Narendra Pub, p 21-38.

Somvanshi, V.S. 2002. Satellite Remote Sensing Applications in Marine Fisheries, *Fishing Chimes* 22(2), p 27-31.

Soto, Doris et al. 2012. Implementing the Ecosystem Approach to Fisheries and Aquaculture. *FAO Aquaculture Newsletter* 49, June 2012.

South Indian Federation of Fishermen Societies. http://www.siffs.org/. [Accessed on 15 Nov 2012].

Sreedhar, U. 2009. Remote Sensing and Fisheries. In: Meenakumari, B. et al. (Eds). *Handbook of Fishing Technology*. Cochin: Central Institute of Fisheries Technology, pp 327-337.

Sreenivasulu, V and Nandwana, H. B. 2001. Networking of Agricultural Information Systems and Services in India., *Inspel.*, 4(1), p 13-15.

Srivastava, U.K. and Dharma Reddy, M. 1983. Fisheries Development in India. New Delhi: Concept Publishing Company.

Srivastava, U.K., Dholakia, B.H., Vathsala, S and Chidambaram, K. 1991. Fishery Sector of India. New Delhi: Oxford & IBH Pub, p 226.

Stallings, William.1988. Data and Computer Communication. 2nd ed. New York: MacMillan.

Stanley, R.D. and Rice, J. 2003. Participatory Research in the British Columbia Groundfish Fishery In: *Fisheries Center Research Reports 11(1) 44-56*. Vancouver BC: University of British Columbia Press.

State Institute of Rural Development. http://www.sird.kerala.gov.in. [Accessed on 14 Nov 2012].

State Resource Centre-Kerala. www.srckerala.org. [Accessed on13Nov 2012].

Subba Rao, N. 1986. Economics of Fisheries. New Delhi: Daya Publishing.

Subbaiah, R. 1985. Conceptual Framework for an Indian National Agricultural Information System (INAGRIS). *PhD Thesis*. Trivandrum: University of Kerala.

Subbaih, A and Umarani, K. 2001. Mapping Agricultural Research in India: A Profile based on CAB Abstracts 1998. *Current Science* 81(8), p 896-906.

Sugunan, V.V. 1995. Reservoir Fisheries of India. *FAO Fisheries Technical Paper 345*. Rome: Food and Agriculture Organization, pp. 423.

Sujatha, H.R. 2007. Use of Electronic Information Sources in Fisheries Science in South India. *Ph D Thesis*, Mangalore: Mangalore University.

Sujatha, H.R. and Mudhol, M.V. 2006. Electronic Information Resources on Fisheries: A study. *Annals of Library and Information Studies* 53, Jun 2006, p 96-102.

Sujatha, H.R. and Mudhol, M.V. 2009. Evaluation of Electronic Information Services in the Fisheries College Libraries in South India: A study. *SRELS Journal of Information Management*. 46 (3), p 277-282.

Sujatha, H.R., Mudhol, M.V.and Murthy.S.H. 2006. Need for a National Fisheries Information System. *SRELS Journal of Information Management* 43(4), p 341-355.

Swaminathan, M.S. 1993. Information Technology: A Dialogue. Chennai: Macmillan.

The Hindu 2009. Fishnet Portal for Coastal States- *News* 12 Jan 2009, Kochi.

Tim, S Gray 2005. Participatory Fisheries Governance. In: Tim, S Gray. (Ed). *Participation in Fisheries Governance*. Dordrecht: Springer.

Turabian, K.L. 1995. A Manual for Writers of Term Papers, Thesis, and Dissertations, 6ed. Chicago: University of Chicago Press.

UGC. 1988. Development of an Information and Library Network: Report of the Inter Agency Working Group. New Delhi: University Grants Commission.

UNESCO. 1979. Inter-Governmental Conference on Scientific and Technological Information for Development, UNISIST-II, Paris, May 28-Jun 1, 1979 (Main Working Document. PGI/UNISIST-II/4.). Paris: UN Educational, Scientific and Cultural Organization.

United Nations. 1987. World Commission on Environment and Development: Our Common Future. Oxford: Oxford University Press.

University of Utah. 2013. Library Regulations [Online]. Available at: http:/ / regulations. Utah.edu/it /4-002.php Definitions. [Accessed on 18 Apr 2013]

Vaas, K.K. 2006. Coldwater fisheries. In: Ayyappan, S et al. (Eds). *Handbook of Fisheries and Aquaculture*. New Delhi: Indian Council of Agricultural Research, p 208-226.

Vaughan, Liwen. 2009. Statistical Methods for the Information Professionals: A Practical Painless Approach to Understanding, Using and Interpreting Statistics. New Delhi: Ess Ess Publications. p1-209.

Venugopal, S. 2005. Aquaculture, Jaipur: Pointer Publishers. pp 53.

Vickery, B and Vickery, A. 1994. Information Science in Theory and Practice. London: Bowker-Saur. p222.

Webster, J.G and Collins, J. 2005. Fisheries Information in Developing Countries, FAO Fisheries Circular No.1006. Rome: Food and Agriculture Organization.

Webster, Noah. 1976. New Twentieth Century Dictionary of the English Language Unabridged 2nd edn. Havana: Collins World.

Wikipedia. 2012 [Online]. Available at: http://en.wikipedia.org/wiki/ List_of_universities[Accessed on 23 Dec 2012].

Wikipedia. 2013 [Online]. Available at: http://en.wikipedia.org/wiki/ WorldCat. [Accessed on 25 Mar 2013].

Wilson, D.C and Delaney, A.E. 2005. Scientific Knowledge and Participation in the Governance of Fisheries in the North Sea. In:

Tim, S Gray. (Ed). *Participation in Fisheries Governance*. Dordrecht: Springer.

World Bank, FAO and WorldFish. 2010. The Hidden Harvest: The Global Contribution of Capture Fisheries. Washington, DC: Agriculture and Rural Development Department, Sustainable Development Network, World Bank.

World Bank. 2008. infoDev: Information for Development Programme.[Online]. Available at: http://www.infodev.org/en/index.html. [Accessed on 07 Jul 2012].

Yellen, J.E. et al. 1995. A Middle Stone-age Worked Bone Industry from Katanda, Upper Semliki Valley, Zaire, *Science* 268: 553-556.

Younis, A.S. and Donaldson, G. 1982. Fishery: Sector Policy Paper. Washington, DC: The World Bank, p 10.

Zoological Survey of India. http://www.zsi.gov.in. [Accessed on 16 Nov 2012].

❑❑❑

Appendices

Appendix 1 (Refer to Chapter 5)

Central Fisheries Institutions of India

Central Institute of Fisheries Nautical and Engineering Training (CIFNET)

HQs: Kochi; RCs; Chennai & Vizag; Control Ministry/Agency: DAHDF, MoA.

Broad Area of Activity: Generation of technical personnel required for manning the large ocean-going fishing vessels and skilled persons for allied industries of marine fisheries.

Info dissemination Products/Media/Methods/Tools: Library, Bulletins, Annual Reports, training programmes, Web Home page.

Library: Yes; Professionals: one; Professional Managerial Head: Nil; Resource Sharing Prog: Nil.

Services offered: Acquisition, Tech Processing, Periodicals, OPAC, Routine Services, Back Volumes.

National Institute of Fisheries Post Harvest Technology and Training (NIFPHATT)

HQs: Kochi; RCs: Nil; Control Min/Agency: DAHDF, MoA.

Broad Area of Activity: Post-harvest technology up-gradation and dissemination.

Info dissemination Products/ Media/Methods/Tools: Newsletters, booklets, training, workshops, consultancy services, Web Home page.

Library: Yes; Professionals: Nil; Professional Managerial Head: Nil; Resource Sharing Prog: Nil

Services offered: Nil

Fishery Survey of India (FSI)

HQs: Mumbai; RCs: Porbandar, Mumbai, Murmugao, Kochi, Chennai, Visakhapatnam and Port Blair ; Control Min/Agency: DAHDF, MoA.

Broad Area of Activity: Survey and assessment of marine fishery resources of the Indian EEZ.

Info dissemination Products/Media/Methods/Tools: Bulletins, charts, atlas, occasional papers, special publications, workshops, Resources Information Series and quarterly newsletter namely *Meena News,* Web Home page.

Library: Nil; Professionals: Nil; Professional Managerial Head: Nil; Resource Sharing Prog: Nil.

Services offered: Nil.

Central Institute of Coastal Engineering for Fishery (CICEF)

HQs: Bangalore; RCs: Nil; Control Min/Agency: DAHDF MoA.

Broad Area of Activity: Conducting engineering and economic investigations and preparing the fisheries harbor projects and brackishwater farms.

Info dissemination Products/Media/Methods/Tools: Web Home page.

Library: Nil; Professionals: Nil; Professional Managerial Head: Nil; Resource Sharing Prog: Nil;

Services offered: Nil.

National Fisheries Development Board (NFDB)

HQs: Hyderabad; RCs: Nil; Control Min/Agency: DAHDF, MoA.

Broad Area of Activity: Extending assistance to the various agencies for implementation of activities under inland, brackish water and marine sectors; act as a platform for bringing together the research and development organizations and stakeholders; provides financial support to create new infrastructure and to modernize the existing infrastructure in public and private sector.

Info dissemination Products/Media/Methods/Tools: Newsletter, Web Home page.

Library: Nil; Professionals: Nil; Professional Managerial Head: Nil; Resource Sharing Prog: Nil.

Services offered: Nil.

Coastal Aquaculture Authority (CAA)

HQs: Chennai; Control Min/Agency: DAHDF, MoA

Broad Area of Activity: Regulating the activities connected with coastal aquaculture and matters connected therewith or incidental thereto.

Info dissemination Products/Media/Methods/Tools: standards, notifications, rules and regulations on coastal aquaculture.

Library: Nil; Professionals: Nil; Professional Managerial Head: Nil; Resource Sharing Prog: Nil

Services offered: Nil

Marine Products Export Development Authority (MPEDA)

HQs: Kochi; RCs: Tokyo, New York, Vizhinjam, Kakinada, Ernakulam.; Control Min/Agency: Min. of Commerce.

Broad Area of Activity: Develop and regulate marine products industry with special reference to export promotion.

Info dissemination Media/Methods/Tools: Newsletter, Directories, Handbooks, Statistics, Web Home page.

Library: Yes; Professionals: One; Professional Managerial Head: Nil; Resource Sharing Prog: Nil.

Services offered: Acquisition, Tech Processing, Periodicals, OPAC, Routine Services,

Current Awareness Service, e-mail alerts, Back Volumes.

Centre for Marine Living Resources and Ecology (CMLRE)

HQs: Kochi; RCs: Nil; Control Min/Agency: Dept. of Ocean Development, Min of Earth Science.

Broad Area of Activity: Coordinating and implementing the Marine Living Resources (MLR) Programme of the Department envisaging survey, assessment and exploitation of the MLR in the Indian EEZ.

Info dissemination Media/Methods/Tools: Web Home page.

Library: Nil Professionals: Nil; Professional Managerial Head: Nil; Resource Sharing Prog : Nil

Services offered: Nil

National Federation of Fishermen's Cooperatives Ltd (FISHCOPFED)

HQs: New Delhi; RCs: Nil; Control Min/Agency: MoA.

Broad Area of Activity: Promotional, welfare, and business.

Info dissemination Media/Methods/Tools: Newsletter.

Library: Nil Professionals: Nil; Professional Managerial Head: Nil; Resource Sharing Prog: Nil Services offered: Nil

Central Inland Capture Fisheries Research Institute (CIFRI)

HQs: Barrackpore; RCs: Allahabad, Bangalore, Vadodara and Guwahati; Control Min/Agency: ICAR.

Broad Area of Activity: Conduct investigation for a proper appraisal of inland fisheries resources on the country and to evolve suitable methods for their conservation and optimum utilization.

Info dissemination Media/Methods/Tools: Bulletins, policy papers, Annual Reports, books, leaflets, Web Home page.

Library: Yes Professionals: 2; Professional Managerial Head: Nil; Resource Sharing Prog: Preparation of Indian Fisheries Abstracts; Services offered: Acquisition, Tech Processing, Periodicals, OPAC, Routine Services, Back volumes.

Central Institute of Fisheries Education (CIFE)

HQs: Mumbai; RCs: Kolkota; Control Min/Agency: (Deemed University) ICAR.

Broad Area of Activity: Develop professionals and human resource; conduct M F Sc and Ph D in specializations.

Info dissemination Media/Methods/Tools: Annual Report, Training, Web Home page.

Library: Yes Professionals: 3; Professional Managerial Head: Nil; Resource Sharing Prog: Content Page Service, Participation in Worldcat/OCLC Programme.

Services offered: Acquisition, Tech Processing, Periodicals, OPAC, Routine Services, Back volumes.

Central Marine Fisheries Research Institute (CMFRI)

HQs: Kochi; RCs: Three plus Eight along the Indian coast; Control Min/Agency: ICAR

Broad Area of Activity: Research and development on capture fisheries and sea farming technologies, transfer of technology and consultancy services.

Info dissemination Media/Methods/Tools: Annual Report, Tech Bulletins, Newsletter, Information Services, Training, Web Home page, Eprints@cmfri.

Library: Yes; Professionals: 5; Professional Managerial Head: Nil; Resource Sharing Prog: Preparation of Marine Information Services;

Services offered: Acquisition, Tech Processing, Periodicals, OPAC, Routine Services, Back volumes, Eprints@cmfri, Database Search, Current Awareness Service, E-mail alerts

Central Institute of Fisheries Technology (CIFT)

HQs: Kochi; RCs: Veraval, Visakhapatanam, Kurla, Mumbai, Calicut and Hoshangabad; Control Min/Agency: ICAR.

Broad Area of Activity: works in technology aspects of production, processing and distribution of fisheries.

Info dissemination Media/Methods/Tools: Training programmes, publications, information services, newsletter, Technology Advisory

Services, Annual Report, Web Home page.

Library: Yes Professionals: Two; Professional Managerial Head: Nil; Resource Sharing Prog: Input centre for ASFA database in India.

Services offered: Acquisition, Tech Processing, Periodicals, OPAC, Routine Services, Back Volumes, Digital Archive, Database Search.

Central Institute of Freshwater Aquaculture (CIFA)

HQs: Bhubaneswar; RCs: Kolkata, Bangalore; Control Min/ Agency: ICAR.

Broad Area of Activity: Conducts research to evolve production technologies in freshwater aquaculture.

Info dissemination Media/Methods/Tools: Publications, Annual Reports, News Letters, trainings, workshops, Web Home page.

Library: Yes Professionals: One; Professional Managerial Head: Nil; Resource Sharing Prog: National depository of FAO (Department of Fisheries and Aquaculture) publications.

Services offered: Acquisition, Tech Processing, Periodicals, OPAC, Routine Services, Back Volumes.

Central Institute of Brackishwater Aquaculture (CIBA)

HQs: Chennai; RCs: Nil; Control Min/Agency: ICAR.

Broad Area of Activity: Nodal institute to cater to the needs of the brackishwater aquaculture sector of the country.

Info dissemination Media/Methods/Tools: Annual Reports, bulletins, training manuals, extension and other miscellaneous publications, Web Home page.

Library: Yes Professionals: One; Professional Managerial Head: Nil; Resource Sharing Prog: Nil

Services offered: Acquisition, Tech Processing, Periodicals, OPAC, Routine Services, Back Volumes.

Directorate of Coldwater Fisheries Research (DCFR)

HQs: Bhimtal.; Control Min/Agency: ICAR.

Broad Area of Activity: Research on coldwater fishery resources; on biology, ecology, breeding, etc. of cold-water fishes.

Info dissemination Media/Methods/Tools: Annual Reports, News Letters, technical bulletins, publications, Web Home page.

Library: Yes Professionals: One; Professional Managerial Head: Nil; Resource Sharing Prog: Nil.

Services offered: Acquisition, Tech Processing, Periodicals, OPAC, Routine Services, Back Volumes.

National Bureau of Fish Genetic Resources (NBFGR)

HQs: Lucknow.; RCs: Kochi.; Control Min/Agency: ICAR

Broad Area of Activity: Conducts work on genetic characterization, gene-banking, biodiversity database and conservation of various fish species.

Info dissemination Media/Methods/Tools: Annual Reports, News Letters, technical bulletins, publications, Web Home page.

Library: Yes Professionals: 3; Professional Managerial Head: Nil; Resource Sharing Prog: Nil.

Services offered: Acquisition, Tech Processing, Periodicals, OPAC, Routine Services, Back Volumes.

Appendix 2 (Refer to Chapter 5)

Universities and Colleges Offering Fisheries Courses

A: Universities/Colleges

No	Institute	University	Bachelor's	Master's	Doctoral
1	**Kerala**KUFOS, Kochi (*formerly* College of Fisheries)	KUFOS, Kochi (*formerly* KAU)	"	"	"
2	**Tamil Nadu** TNFU, Nagapattinam(formed in 2012). FCRI, Tuticorin and IFT, Ponneri and Nagapattinam are the constituent institutions.				
3	**Deemed Central University** CIFE, Mumbai	ICAR,New Delhi	-	"	"
4	**Andhra Pradesh** CoFSc, Muthukur, Nellore-524344	SVUTTirupathi	"	"	-
5	**Assam** CoFSc, Raha-782103	AAU, Jorhat	"	"	-
6	**Bihar**CoF, Tirhut, Muzaffarpur, Pusa Road, Dholi	RajendraAgril Univ, Samastipur	"	-	-
7	**Chattisgarh** CoF, Kawardha, Kabirdham Dist	IGKVV,Raipur	"	-	-
8	**Gujarat**CoFSc, Veraval-362265	JAU, Junagadh	"	"	-
9	**Jammu & Kashmir** CoF, Srinagar-190006	SKUAST-K, Srinagar	"	"	-
10	**Karnataka** CoF, Mangalore-575002	KVAFSUBidar-585401	"	"	"
11	**Maharashtra** CoF, Ratnagiri-415629	Dr BSKKV, Dapoli	"	"	-
12	MaharashtraCoF, Nagpur	MAFSU,Nagpur	"	-	-
13	MaharashtraCoFSc, Udgir	MAFSU,Nagpur	"	-	-
14	**Odisha** CoF, Rangailunda, Ganjam, Berhampur-760007	OUAT, Bhubaneswar	"	"	-

15	**Punjab** CoF, Ludhiana-141004	GADVASU, Ludhiana	"	"	-
16	**Rajastan** CoF, Udaipur -313001	MPUAT, Udaipur	"	"	-
17	**Tamil Nadu** FCRI, Tuticorin-628008	TNFU Nagapatinam	"	"	"
18	**Tripura** CoF, Lembucherra, Agarthala	CAU, Lamphelpat, Imphal	"	"	-
19	**Uttar Pradesh** CoF, Kumarganj, Faizabad	NDUAT, Lucknow	"	-	-
20	**Uttarkhand** CoFSc, Pantnagar-263145	GBPUAT, Pant Nagar	"	"	"
21	**West Bengal** Faculty of Fisheries Science, 5 Budherhat Rd, Panchasayar-PO, Chakgaria Campus, Kolkota-700094	WBUAFS, Kolkata	"	"	"

B: Specialized/Allied Courses

No.	Institution	Course	Subjects
1	KUFOS, Kochi	MBA LLM M Tech M Sc MFSc	Fisheries/Rural Management Maritime Law ICZ Management Physical, Biological Oceanography Remote Sensing, Geo Sciences, Food Science, Applied StatisticsAll Branches of fisheries andAquatic Animal Health Management, Fisheries Engineering, Nutrition, Feed Technology etc
2	Faculty of Marine Sciences, CUSAT, Kochi, Kerala.	M Sc; Ph D	Industrial Fisheries, Marine Geology, Marine Biologyand Oceanography
3	IIT, Kharagpur	M Tech Ph D	Aquaculture Engineering
4	College of Engineering, Waltair	BE	Fishery Engineering
5	TIFR, Mumbai	M Sc	Marine Geo-chemistry

6	CASABF, Kerala University, Trivandrum	M Sc M Phil Ph D	Fisheries and Aquatic Biology
7	CASMB, Parangipettai Annamalai University Tamil Nadu	M Sc	Marine Biology
8	Andhra University, Vishakapatnam	M Sc	Fishery Science; Coastal Aquaculture andMarine Biotechnology, Marine Geology; Marine Biology
9	Affiliated Colleges. MG University, Kottayam	B Sc M Sc	AquacultureIndustrial Fish & FisheriesApplied Fisheries and Aquaculture Aquaculture & Fish Processing
10	Affiliated Colleges. University of Kerala. Trivandrum.	M Sc	Zoology (Fisheries)
11	SelfFinancing College. Calicut University, Calicut	M Sc	Fisheries
12	NIT-Karnataka, Suratkal, Mangalore	Diploma	Fish Harbour Engineering
13	Madras Christian College, Chennai-600059 affiliated to University of MadrasDept of Marine Studiesand Coastal Resource Management.	PG Diploma	Coastal Aquaculture Course imparted by
14	Indian Institute of Foreign Trade, New Delhi	Diploma	International Trade in Seafood Industry
15	Acharya Nagarjuna University, Guntur	M Sc	Aquaculture
16	Barkatullah Universtiy, Bhopal	M Sc	Applied Aquaculture
17	Suganthi Devadason Marine Research Inst, Tuticorin, and Centre for Marine Sciences and Technology, Tirunalveli. Affiliated to Manon-manian Sundarnar University, Tirunalveli-629502, Tamil Nadu	MSc, MPhil, Ph DPG Diploma	Marine Fisheries

Appendix 3 (Refer to Chapter 5)

Fisheries Out Stream Institutions, Programmes, NGOs, Associations and Societies

A: Major Out Stream Fisheries Institutions in India

Zoological Survey of India (ZSI)

HQs: Kolkota; RCs: In different parts of India; Control Min/ Agency:Min. of Environment, Forests and Climate Change.

Broad Area of Activity: Taxonomic study of all kinds of animals from Protozoa to Mammalia, occurring in all possible habitats.

Info dissemination Products/Media/Methods/Tools: News Letter, ZSI Holdings, Checklist of Indian Fauna and Faunal Resource Table, Web Home Page.

Library & Information Division: Library at HQs has rich collections in zoological literature with Web OPAC

National Institute of Oceanography (NIO)

HQs: Goa; RCs: Kochi, Mumbai, Vizag; Control Min/Agency: CSIR

Broad Area of Activity: R&D support for utilizing the ocean resources and to develop technologies necessary for exploiting the ocean resources.

Info dissemination Products/Media/Methods/Tools: Publications, Newsletter, Web Portal.

Library & Information Division: Notable collection of printed literature on ocean sciences in the country. Recognized as the National Information Centre for Marine Science (NICMAS) and also acts as the ASFA centre, monitoring the literature on aquatic sciences published in the Indian Journals and other sources. Member of IAMSLIC. Part of IAMSLIC Z39.50 Distributed Library. Resource sharing programme. Part of National Ocean Information System (NOIS).

Indian National Centre for Ocean Information System (INCOIS)

HQs: Hyderabad; Control Min/Agency: MoES.

Broad Area of Activity: Central repository for marine data in India. Provide information on physical, chemical, biological and geological parameters of ocean and coasts on spatial and temporal domains.

Info dissemination Products/Media/Methods/Tools: Newsletter, Annual Reports, Web Portal, Electronic Bulletin Board. Services provided by INCOIS comprise of Potential Fishing Zone (PFZ); Ocean State Forecast (OSF); Marine Meteorological Advisory Services; Web-based Ocean Information Services; Climate / Monsoon / Weather Forecast; Monitoring of Pollution / Oil Spill and Global Ocean Observing System. Designated as the National Oceanographic Data Centre by the International Oceanographic Commission (IOC). Serve as the National Argo Data Centre; Regional Argo Data Centre; Regional Data Centre and clearing house for the Indian Ocean region.

Library & Information Division: Resources on the frontier areas of ocean science, geophysics and allied sciences in print and electronic formats.

National Institute of Ocean Technology (NIOT)

HQs: Chennai.; RCs: Nil.; Control Min/Agency: MoES.

Broad Area of Activity: To develop reliable indigenous technology to solve various engineering problems associated with harvesting of non-living and living resources in the Indian EEZ

Info dissemination Products/Media/Methods/Tools: Annual Report, Training, Web Page.

Library & Information Division: Collections pertaining to the areas of activity of the institute.

Central Food Technological Research Institute (CFTRI)

HQs: Mysore; RCs: Bangalore, Hyderabad, Lucknow and Mumbai.; Control Min/Agency: CSIR

Broad Area of Activity: Knowledge generation in food biotechnology, microbiology, sensory science and food safety

Info dissemination Products/Media/Methods/Tools: Training, Annual Report, Newsletter, Web Home Page.

Library & Information Division: Serves the R&D community to keep track of the technological advances worldwide in food science and technology. Provide access to global information, databases and e-journals through CSIR Consortium and high bandwidth Internet. Current Awareness Service; Document Delivery Service; National and International Database Search Service, apart from routine library services.

National Institute of Nutrition (NIN)

HQs: Hyderabad.; Control Min/Agency: Min. of Health & Family Welfare/ICMR

Broad Area of Activity: Food and nutrition research, with special reference to protein energy malnutrition

Info dissemination Products/Media/Methods/Tools: Publishes gratis material on nutrition, conducts integrated nutrition education camps, produce educational aids, instructional CDs, TV films and exhibits museum, Web Home Page.

Library & Information Division: Poly-media based Information Centre with resources in health and nutrition.

National Remote Sensing Agency (NRSA)

HQs: Hyderabad.; Control Min/Agency: Department of Space

Broad Area of Activity: Receiving and distributing remote sensing data for applications like Natural Resource Management, Disaster Management and Geographical Information Management. NRSA's data is used by a number of agencies of the Government of India in the areas of ground water targeting, flood mapping, water resource mapping, soil mapping, watershed management, crop estimation, ocean studies, etc.

Info dissemination Products/Media/Methods/Tools: Training, India-Water Resources Information System (WRIS), Integrated Water Resources Management (IWRM). Web Portal.

Library & Information Division: Serves the R&D community to keep track of the technological advances worldwide in Remote Sensing. Offer Current Awareness Service; Document Delivery Service; National and International Database Search Service apart from routine library services.

Indian Agricultural Research Institute (IARI)

HQs: New Delhi.; RCs: Nil.; Control Min/Agency: ICAR.

Broad Area of Activity: Premier national institute for agricultural research, education and extension. Besides basic research, applied and commodity research also conducted on major crops

Info dissemination Products/Media/Methods/Tools: Annual Report, Newsletter, Web Home Page.

Library & Information Division: Largest agro-biological libraries in South-East Asia housing six lakh documents belonging to agricultural science. Depository of FAO, International Development Research Centre (IDRC), Asian Vegetable Research and Development Center (AVRDC) and CGIAR publications.

Indian Agricultural Statistics Research Institute (IASRI)

HQs: New Delhi; RCs: Nil; Control Min/Agency: ICAR.

Broad Area of Activity: Conducting basic, applied and adaptive research in agricultural statistics and computer application and to disseminate knowledge and information produced.

Info dissemination Products/Media/Methods/Tools: Training, Web Home Page

Library & Information Division : Resource base in the field of Agricultural Statistics, Computer Applications and allied fields.

National Academy of Agricultural Research Management (NAARM)

HQs: Hyderabad; RCs: Nil; Control Min/Agency: ICAR

Broad Area of Activity: To enhance the performance of India's National Agricultural Research System through research, capacity strengthening and policy support in agricultural research and education management.

Info dissemination Products/Media/Methods/Tools: Training, Annual Report, Newsletter, Web Page.

Library & Information Division : Resources on management and agricultural subjects.

National Institute of Agricultural Extension Management (MANAGE)

HQs: Hyderabad; RCs: Nil; Control Min/Agency: ICAR.

Broad Area of Activity: To set up professionalism, guidance and training in agriculture sector warranted by the policies of liberalization and globalization of the economy; sophistication of agricultural technologies, etc.

Info dissemination Products/Media/Methods/Tools: Extension trainings, Annual Report, Newsletter, Web Home page.

Library & Information Division: Resources on Agricultural Extension.

National Centre for Agricultural Economics and Policy Research (NCAP)

HQs: New Delhi; RCs: Nil.; Control Min/Agency: ICAR

Broad Area of Activity: Undertakes research in agricultural economics and policy analysis in technology policy, sustainable agriculture, market and trade, institutional change and growth and modeling in agriculture with a view to strengthen agricultural economics research.

Info dissemination Products/Media/Methods/Tools: Publications, Web Home Page, Training Programmes.

Library & Information Division : Resources such as Statistical Abstracts, Economic Survey, Agricultural census, Input surveys, Livestock census, National Sample Survey, Central Statistical Origanisation and other Government of India publications. Depository of FAO and CGIAR publications

NIRD&Panchayati Raj

HQs: Hyderabad; RCs: Ten .; Control Min/Agency: Ministry of Rural Development.

Broad Area of Activity: examine and analyze the factors contributing to the improvement of economic and social well-being of people in rural areas; to facilitate the rural development efforts with particular emphasis and focus on the rural poor by improving the knowledge, skills and attitudes of rural development officials and non-officials.

Info dissemination Products/Media/Methods/Tools: Training, Workshops, Seminars, Annual Report, Newsletter, Web Home Page.

Library & Information Division: National Resource centre on rural development.

Central Agricultural Research Institute (CARI)

HQs: Andaman and Nicobar Islands; RCs:Nil; Control Min/Agency: ICAR.

Broad Area of Activity: To develop the island agricultural production technologies without affecting the fragile ecosystem of the islands. Division of Fisheries Science focus on the issues related to aquaculture, capture fisheries resources and impact of climate change on coastal bio-resources.

Info dissemination Products/Media/Methods/Tools: Annual Report, Web Home Page.

Library & Information Division: Resources in agriculture, natural resource management, animal sciences, biotechnology, fisheries science and social sciences

Krishi Vigyan Kendras (KVKs) (Fisheries)

HQs: -; RCs: 31 in different parts of India including Lakshadweep; Control Min/Agency: ICAR

Broad Area of Activity: Information Dissemination

Info dissemination Products/Media/Methods/Tools: Training, Testing Laboratory facilities, Demonstration Units, circulation of Technical bulletin, Package of practices etc.

Library & Information Division: Nil

Indian Institute of Packaging (IIP)

HQs: Mumbai.; RCs: Delhi, Kolkata ; Control Min/Agency: Min. of Commerce & Industry

Broad Area of Activity: To attend to the needs on packaging both for domestic and export markets.

Info dissemination Products/Media/Methods/Tools: Advanced Courses, Training, Annual Report, Web Home Page, Exhibitions.

Library & Information Division : Besides documents, collection include packaging related national and international standards on materials, methods and systems, testing and quality control, etc.

Indian Institute of Foreign Trade (IIFT)

HQs: New Delhi.; RCs: Kolkota; Control Min/Agency: Deemed University

Broad Area of Activity: To professionalize the country's foreign trade management and to increase exports by developing human resources, generating, analyzing and disseminating data and conducting research. Conduct surveys on market, trade and tariff, export costs, export benefits, shipping and transport, financing etc.

Info dissemination Products/Media/Methods/Tools: Master courses and advance courses in international business and export management, Annual Report, Newsletter, Web page.

Library & Information Division: Publications of FAO, International Monetary Fund (IMF), Organisation for Economic Co-operation and Development (OECD), United Nations Conference on Trade and Development (UNCTAD), United Nations Centre on Transnational Corporations (UNCTC), World Bank, WTO and other international agencies form the unique reference source in the library.

Export Inspection Council of India (EIC)

HQs: New Delhi; RCs: Mumbai, Kolkata, Kochi and Chennai .; Control Min/Agency: Min. of Commerce & Industry.

Broad Area of Activity: India's official export certification body. An advisory body to the Central Government assisting in to notify commodities, establish standards of quality and to specify type of quality control of such commodities prior to export.

Info dissemination Products/Media/Methods/Tools: QC Inspections carried out by Export Inspection Agencies functioning at Mumbai, Kolkota, Kochi and Chennai.

Library & Information Division (HQs): Documents pertaining to the national and international standards, rules, regulation etc on Quality Control and related aspects.

B: Programmes, NGOs and Associations of National Standing

Bay of Bengal Programme -Inter-Governmental Programme

Main executing agency: FAO; Focal point: DAHFD, MoA; Secretariat: Chennai.

Broad Area of Activity: Mandated to enhance cooperation among member-countries, other countries and organizations in the region of Bay of Bengal by providing technical and management advisory services for socio-ecologically responsible marine fisheries development and management in the region.

Info dissemination Products/Media/Methods/Tools: Publication of working papers, reports, mimeographs, video films and CD-ROMs

Library & Information Division : -Nil

Aquaculture Foundation of India (AFI)

HQs: Chennai.

Broad Area of Activity: Promotion of aquaculture all over India

Info dissemination Products/Media/Methods/Tools: Publications, seminars, workshops, Ocean Life Expo.

Library & Information Division :-Nil

M S Swaminathan Research Foundation (MSSRF)

HQs: Chennai

Broad Area of Activity: Works on the issues of access to communications for poor village communities.

Info dissemination Products/Media/Methods/Tools: Training, awareness programme to the rural poor. Setting up VRCs and VKCs to provide need-based locale-specific, demand-driven information content.

Library & Information Division : HQs.

Seafood Exporters Association of India (SEAI)

HQs: Kochi.; RCs: Eight (in East and West Coast States)

Broad Area of Activity: To protect and promote the interest of the companies engaged in the seafood business and to develop the international trade of seafood from India

Info dissemination Products/Media/Methods/Tools: Publications, Journal, Web Home page.

Library & Information Division : -Nil

C. Organizations for Aquatic Environment Protection, Coastal Management etc.

1. SD Marine Biological Research Institute, Sagar Island, Sundarbans, W Bengal.
2. Brackish Water Research Center, Olpad, Surat, Gujrat.
3. Society of Integrated Coastal Management (SICOM), 9 Institutional Area, Lodhi Road, New Delhi.
4. National Centre for Sustainable Coastal Management (NCSCM), Anna University Campus, Chennai.

D. Learned Societies: Learned Societies fostering Fisheries Science and allied sciences that publish scholarly journals, handbooks, manuals, etc. and conduct seminars/symposia/ workshops:-

1. Asiatic Society, Kolkota (Library is the glory and honour of the society)
2. Bombay Natural History Society, Mumbai (The society has India's oldest and largest natural history library)
3. Indian Fisheries Association, Taraporewala Aquarium, Mumbai : Publishes Journal of Indian Fisheries Association. (Association owns the oldest aquarium in India. Hosts marine and freshwater fishes)
4. Inland Fisheries Society of India, C/o CIFRI, Barrackpore: Dedicated to promoting the cause of inland fisheries in the country.
5. Indian Society of Ichthyologist, C/o ZSI, Santhome High Road, Chennai: Publishes Bulletin '*Matsya*'.
6. Indian Meteorological Society, C/o IMD Lodi Road, New Delhi.
7. Marine Biological Association of India, C/o CMFRI, Kochi: Foster marine biological research in Asia-Pacific.
8. Seaweed Research and Utilisation Association of India, Mandapam, Ramnad Dist, Tamil Nadu.
9. Society of Fishery Technologists C/o CIFT, Kochi.

Appendix 4 (Refer to Chapter 6)

Fisheries Institutions and Agencies of Development in Kerala State

A: Socio-Economic Development Agencies (Fisheries Department, Government of Kerala)

Fish Farmer's Development Agency (FFDA)

HQs: district level agency. RCs: 14 in all the districts

Core Activity: Development of fresh water fish culture by providing funds, extension and infrastructure

Information Dissemination Mode/Media: Conventional, Query with Agency

Library and Information Resources & Services: Nil.

Fisheries Resource Management Society (FIRMA)

HQs: Ernakulam, RCs: Nil

Core Activity: Undertakes projects for the development of fisheries sector with emphasis on management and conservation

Information Dissemination Mode/Media: Conventional, Query with Agency

Library and Information Resources & Services: Nil.

Agency for Development of Aquaculture, Kerala (ADAK)

HQs: Trivandrum. RCs: Alapuzha and Ernakulam

Core Activity: Implement various programmes for the promotion of aquaculture

Information Dissemination Mode/Media: Conventional, Query with Agency

Library and Information Resources & Services: Nil.

Society for Assistance to Fisher Women (SAF)

HQs: Kadungallur; RCs:Nil

Core Activity: Takes up various schemes to encourage and strengthen locally organised social organisation among fisherwomen in coastal areas.

Information Dissemination Mode/Media: Conventional, Query with Agency and Training

Library and Information Resources & Services: Nil.

Marine Enforcement Department (MED)

HQs:Trivandrum RCs: Vizhinjam, Neendakara, Vypin, Beypore and Kannur.

Core Activity: Enforce the provisions contained in Kerala Marine Fishing Regulation Act 1980 (KMFRA) and other regulations in the fisheries sector

Information Dissemination Mode/Media: Nil

Library and Information Resources & Services: Nil.

Kerala State Coastal Area Development Corporation (KSCADC)

HQs:Trivandrum RCs: Nil

Core Activity: Coastal and fisheries infrastructure development, ensuring utilization of harvested resources, socio-economic development of fishermen, technology acquisition, mobilization of financial resources, commercialization and consultancy

Information Dissemination Mode/Media: Nil

Library and Information Resources & Services: Nil.

Kerala Fishermen's Welfare Fund Board (KFWFB)

HQs: Thrissur RCs: Trivandrum, Alleppey, Ernakulam, Kozhikode and Kannur

Core Activity: Implement welfare schemes aimed at providing assistance and relief measures to the fishermen, allied workers and their family at distress

Information Dissemination Mode/Media: Conventional, Query with Agency

Library and Information Resources & Services: Nil.

Kerala State Co-operative Federation for Fisheries Development Ltd (*Matsyafed*)

HQs: Trivandrum RCs: Ten District Offices

Core Activity: Carries out activities for promoting production, procurement, processing and marketing of fish and fishery products for the development of fishermen community. *Matsyafed* is the apex federation of 654 primary Fisherman Co-Operative Societies spread over 10 districts of Kerala, 340 in marine sector, 183 in the inland sector and 131 women co-operatives.

Information Dissemination Mode/Media: Newsletter in Malayalam, Conventional communication links between primary societies and *Matsyafed*

Library and Information Resources & Services: Nil. Extension and mass communication in *Matsyafed* headed by an officer on DGM rank

National Institute of Fisheries Administration and Management (NIFAM)

HQs: Ernakulam. RCs: Nil

Core Activity: Training to personnel of Departments like Local Self Government, Revenue, Survey, Fire Force, Police, Technical Education and *Kudumbasree*, On Job Training for VHSC students, etc.

Information Dissemination Mode/Media: Conventional

Library and Information Resources & Services: Nil

B: Universities and Colleges Offering Fisheries Courses

Kerala University of Fisheries and Ocean Studies (KUFOS)

HQs: Panangad, Kochi; RCs: Puduvype, Thiruvallam

Governance/Administration: Government of Kerala

Core Activity: Offers bachelor, master and doctoral programme in fisheries and related subjects.

Information Dissemination Mode/Media: Newsletter, Web Home page

Library and Information Division Resources, Services & Functions: Acquisition, Tech Processing, Periodicals, OPAC, Back Volumes, databases and e-journals. Library services, resources and infrastructure need up-gradation to a university library system.

Faculty of Marine Science, School of Ocean Science and Technology; School of Industrial Fisheries, Kochi

Governance/Administration: Cochin University of Science and Technology

Core Activity: Imparting education, training and research facilities in basic and applied aspects of ocean science, ocean technology and industrial fisheries.

Information Dissemination Mode/Media: Publications, Journal, News Bulletin, Faculty Library

Library and Information Division Resources, Services & Functions: Acquisition, Tech Processing, Periodicals, OPAC, Back Volumes, Search Services, Routine Services.

Web page of the central library provide links to web OPAC, e-gateway to the Indian Universities, colleges, e-journals, JCCC-UGC Infonet, INDEST-AICTE, SciFinder and *Dyuthi*, the ETD of the University.

Centre of Advanced Study in Aquatic Biology and Fisheries (Dept. of Aquatic Biology and Fisheries (DABF), University of Kerala

HQs:. Karyavattom.

Governance/Administration: University of Kerala, Trivandrum

Core Activity: Offers M Sc, M Phil and Ph D courses in Aquatic Biology and Fisheries

Information Dissemination Mode/Media: Web Page of the University of Kerala

Library and Information Division Resources, Services & Functions: Acquisition, Tech Processing, Periodicals, OPAC, Back Volumes, Search Services, Routine Services

School of Applied Life Sciences (SALS)

HQs: Pathanamthitta

Governance/Administration: Mahatma Gandhi (MG) University, Kottayam

Core Activity: Offers M.Sc. and M Phil degrees in Fishery Biology and Aquaculture under Self-Financing Scheme

Information Dissemination Mode/Media: Nil

Library and Information Division Resources, Services & Functions: Conventional

Colleges Affiliated to the University of Kerala

Fatima Mata National College, Kollam and Sree Narayana College, Cherthala offer M Sc degree course in zoology with specialization in fisheries.

Colleges Affiliated to the MG University

St Albert's College, Ernakulam offer B Sc Industrial Fish and Fisheries and M Sc Aquaculture. Sacred Heart College, Kochi offers Masters Degree in Aquaculture and Fish Processing (under Self Financing scheme)

Colleges Affiliated to the Calicut University

MES Ponnani College, the self financing centre affiliated to the Calicut University conducts MSc in Aquaculture and Fisheries Microbiology.

C: Out Stream Institutions

Kerala Agricultural University (KAU)

HQs: Thrissur. RCs: 6 colleges, 15 research stations, 6 Regional Agricultural Research Stations, 4 Instructional Farms, 7 KVKs, one Central Training Institute, an Academy for Climate Change Education and Research, and Central Library with IT facilities. Veterinary and Fisheries universities have been formed in the year 2010 and 2011 respectively by carving out constituent colleges.

Governance/Administration: Government of Kerala.

Core Activity: Provide the technology, skill and human resources for the scientific improvement of agriculture in the State. Impart agricultural education, research, extension and Transfer of technology

Information Dissemination Mode/Media: Web OPAC, Web Home Page, Newsletter. Central Library as the repository of dissertations, databases, foreign journals and documents in Agriculture and allied subjects.

Library and Information Division Resources, Services & Functions: Acquisition, Tech Processing, Periodicals, OPAC, Back Volumes, Online database and e-journal Search, Routine Services.

Regional Agricultural Research Station (RARS)

HQs: Kumarakom. RCs: RARS is one of RCs of KAU

Governance/Administration: Kerala Agricultural University, Thrissur.

Core Activity: Conducts research on integrated farming systems incorporating crops, livestock and fish; selection of species and their culture for aquaculture in *Kari* lands of Kuttanad; fish culture in cage and pen enclosures in Vembanad lake; fish diseases and their possible relation to aquatic pollution with special reference to Kuttanad; rearing of freshwater prawn in freshwater bodies of Kuttanad, etc.

Information Dissemination Mode/Media: Training, Workshops, Web page of the University

Library and Information Division Resources, Services & Functions: Nil.

Fisheries Research Station (FRS)

HQs: Puthuvypu. RCs: One of the RC of KUFOS

Governance/Administration: Kerala University of Fisheries and Ocean Studies

Core Activity: Fish culture and maintain the estuarine parts, the natural habitat of fishes for their breeding and growth.

Information Dissemination Mode/Media: Training and Demonstrations

Library and Information Division Resources, Services & Functions: Nil

Centre for Development Studies (CDS)

HQs: Trivandrum

Governance/Administration: Government of Kerala

Core Activity: Cutting edge research in applied economics and topics germane to socio-economic development. Fisheries economics is a major area of study by CDS.

Information Dissemination Mode/Media: Training, Workshops, Web Homepage, Library

Library and Information Division Resources, Services & Functions: library is a major repository for social science research with rich resources. collection of books, journals, and publications of national and international research institutes and government. Acquisition, Tech Processing, Periodicals, OPAC, Back Volumes, Online databases, Routine Services.

National Centre for Earth Sciences Studies (NCESS) (*Formerly Centre for Earth Sciences Studies-CESS)*

Control Agency: MoES

HQs: Trivandrum. RCs: Nil

Governance/Administration: Govt. of India (Formerly Govt. of Kerala)

Core Activity: Conduct researches and studies related to the Earth System especially Earth System Dynamics and Earth Science Applications

Information Dissemination Mode/Media: Publications, Annual Reports, Newsletter, research updates, Research publications, Library with comprehensive resources on the subject, Web Page, Nodal Dissemination Centre of Ocean Warning in the regional language for Kerala coast.

Library and Information Division Resources, Services & Functions: Resource Rich. Acquisition, Tech Processing, Periodicals, OPAC, Back Volumes, Online databases, Routine Services

Centre for Water Resources Development and Management (CWRDM)

HQs: Kozhikode. RCs: Nil

Governance/Administration: Government of Kerala

Core Activity: Research and development in the sphere of water management

Information Dissemination Mode/Media: Annual Report, Newsletter, Library, Web page

Library and Information Division Resources, Services & Functions: Documents on water resources and allied areas. Acquisition, Tech Processing, Periodicals, OPAC, Back Volumes, Routine Services

Kerala Forest Research Institute (KFRI)

HQs: Peechi. RCs: Nil

Governance/Administration: Government of Kerala

Core Activity: Provide scientific support for decision making on matters related to forestry, with particular emphasis on conservation, sustainable utilization and scientific management of natural resources. Ecosystem and landscape analysis, rehabilitation and restoration, population ecology, biodiversity evaluation and conservation of fragile ecosystems, traditional knowledge system analysis and biodiversity-informatics, inventorisation of biodiversity of different forest types and protected areas, evaluation of below-ground biodiversity, taxonomic studies and conservation of flora

Information Dissemination Mode/Media: Annual Report, Newsletter, Web Page, Library

Library and Information Division Resources, Services & Functions: Resource centre on tropical forestry. Special repository of literature on teak, bamboo and rattan. National level Bamboo Information Centre. Routine Services, Acquisition, Tech Processing, Periodicals, Back Volumes, OPAC, Databases.

Council for Food Research and Development (CFRD)

HQs: Konni.

RCs: Runs College of Indigenous Food Technology, Konni a Self Finance College affiliated to M.G. University, Kottayam

Governance/Administration: Government of Kerala

Core Activity: Research in indigenous food and food technology

Information Dissemination Mode/Media: Nil

Library and Information Division Resources, Services & Functions: Conventional

Kerala Institute for Entrepreneurship Development (KIED)

HQs: Kalamassery.

Governance/Administration: Government of Kerala

Core Activity: Promotion and development of entrepreneurial activities in the State

Information Dissemination Mode/Media: Programmes on any production related entrepreneurship development

Library and Information Division Resources, Services & Functions: Nil

Kerala Rural Employment and Welfare Society (KREWS)

HQs: Trivandrum.

Governance/Administration: Government of Kerala

Core Activity: implement schemes designed to promote the progress and welfare of the rural people and to improve the employment potential for the young men and women of the rural areas

Information Dissemination Mode/Media: Conventional.

Library and Information Division Resources, Services & Functions: Nil

State Institute of Rural Development (SIRD)

HQs: Kottarakkara

Governance/Administration: Government of Kerala

Core Activity: Developing managerial skills, organizational abilities, leadership qualities and decision making skills among different categories of government officials, elected representatives of Panchayats and members of NGOs who are engaged in rural developmental activities in the State of Kerala

Information Dissemination Mode/Media: Conventional

Library and Information Division Resources, Services & Functions: Has resources on rural development, poverty alleviation, decentralized planning, women development, management, entrepreneurship development, etc. Routine services.

State Resource Centre-Kerala (SRC-K)

HQs: Trivandrum. RCs: Nil.

Governance/Administration: General Education Department, Government of Kerala

Core Activity: providing academic and technical resource support to all the agencies in the state engaged in adult and continuing education programmes

Information Dissemination Mode/Media: Conventional.

Library and Information Division Resources, Services & Functions: Nil

D: NGOs, Associations and Societies

Centre for Fisheries Studies (CFS)

NGO. HQs: Trivandrum

Area of Activity: Function as research, documentation and information centre and to network with the researchers, NGOs, Government agencies and academic institutions relevant to fisheries sector. CFS conducts researches on issues of fisheries sector and proposes means and ways to rectify them.

Info dissemination Products/Media/Methods/Tools: Training, awareness programmes. Organize and promote new fishermen societies in fishing villages in Trivandrum District

Library & Information Division : Rich resources especially on social issues. Subscribe to newspapers, popular magazines, periodicals and newsletters related to fisheries and socio-cultural aspects. News paper cutting service and its documentation on the subjects of Aquarium Fish, Coastal zone issues, Port issues, Fish and Fisheries, Scholarship and Education Policy Making, Fishermen Development Programme, etc.

Malabar Coastal Institute for Training, Research and Action (MCITRA)

NGO. HQs: Kozhikkode

Area of Activity: Developing a knowledge base through research studies, dissemination of the research findings, training of different stakeholders of the coastal communities, networking and collaboration in direct development and socio-political action.

Info dissemination Products/Media/Methods/Tools: Research studies, training programs, networking with various agencies, publishes the research reports, dossiers, leaflets, newsletters, policy analysis papers and posters.

Library & Information Division : Rich in scientifically documented materials on social and developmental issues related to fisheries, agriculture, environment, women, children, government policies, international agreements, etc.

Kerala Institute for Environment and Development (KIED)

NGO. HQs: Trivandrum

Area of Activity: Voluntary organization of scientists, researchers, professionals, and extension workers concerned with the promotion of development that is socially, economically and environmentally sustainable. Undertake research activities on development and environment, develop appropriate methodologies for research, and impart trainings for researchers and social workers.

Info dissemination Products/Media/Methods/Tools: Training, awareness programmes

Library & Information Division : Resources on developmental and environmental sciences

South Indian Federation of Fishermen Societies (SIFFS)

HQs : Trivandrum. RCs : Calicut, Kakinada, Mangalore, Tranquebar and Rameshwaram

Area of Activity: Establish producer control over fish marketing and inputs, basically to liberate fishermen from the clutches of middlemen, merchants and money lenders

Info dissemination Products/Media/Methods/Tools: Awareness programmes, providing credit for renewal of fishing equipment and promoting savings.

Library & Information Division : Village Information Centre in Trivandrum deploying ICT facilities.

Appendix 5 (Refer to Chapters 4 and 10)

International Institutions and Resources of Fisheries Information

Aquaculture Network Information Centre (AquaNIC) : AquaNIC houses or provides links to thousands of state, national, and international aquaculture publications, newsletters, visual media, calendars, job services, directories and specialty sections for species and production systems. The goals of AquaNIC are to (1) provide access to all electronic information at the national and international level, and (2) increase the quantity and quality of electronic information available to the aquaculture industry. Source: [Online]. Available at: http://aquanic.org/

Bay of Bengal Large Marine Ecosystem (BOBLME) : Bangladesh, India, Indonesia, Malaysia, Maldives, Myanmar, Sri Lanka, and Thailand are collaborating through the Bay of Bengal Large Marine Ecosystem (BOBLME) Project to better the lives of their coastal populations by improving regional management of the Bay of Bengal environment and its fisheries. Source : [Online]. Available at: http://www.boblme.org/

Centre for Environment, Fisheries and Aquaculture (CEFAS) :CEFAS works towards healthy and sustainable marine and freshwater environments by collecting, managing and interpreting environmental, biodiversity and fisheries data. Source: [Online]. Available at: http://www.cefas.defra.gov.uk

Centre for Maritime Research (MARE) :MARE is an interdisciplinary social-science network organization interested in the use and management of marine resources. Its objective is to provide a stimulating intellectual climate for academics and policymakers in Europe as well as in the South. Although MARE limits its action radius to the social sciences, it seeks active collaboration with other disciplines. It strives to maintain a balanced mix of academic and policy-oriented research. MARE takes a global perspective, emphasizing the coastal zones of Europe, Asia, and Africa. It covers a broad spectrum of topics, drawing on expertise from fields such as law, history, economics, political science, public administration, anthropology, and geography. Source: [Online]. Available at: :http://www.mare

Centre for Natural Resource Economics and Policy (CNREP) : CNREP helps meeting the challenge of reconciling the duel needs for economic viability and environmental integrity by improving the management and allocation of the natural resources. The centre considers fisheries as one of the natural capital assets to be managed efficiently for both current and future generations. Source: [Online]. Available at: http://www.cnrep.lsu.edu/

Coral Reef Targeted Research and Capacity Building for Management (CRTR): CRTR Program is a leading international coral reef research initiative that provides a coordinated approach to credible, factual and scientifically-proven knowledge for improved coral reef management. An impressive resource for coral reef researchers, managers and policy makers is accessible by visiting publications and tools on the web page. Source: [Online]. Available at: http://www.gefcoral.org

Danish Institute of Fisheries Research (DIFRES): The research institute produces information for use in management of living resources of fish and shellfish in the sea and participates in the international cooperative research. Source: [Online]. Available at: :http://www.aqua.dtu.dk/English.aspx

FISH INFONetwork (FIN): FIN consists of seven independent intergovernmental organisations as well as FAO GLOBEFISH. The network provides services to private industry and to governments particularly in developing countries and countries in transition. Execution of multilateral and bilateral projects is one of the main activities of the network. INFOPESCA (South and Central America), INFOFISH (Asia and Pacific region), INFOPECHE (Africa), INFOSA (Southern African sub-office of INFOPECHE), INFOSAMAK (Arab countries), EUROFISH (Eastern and Central Europe) and INFOYU (China) are the individual services of FIN. Source: [Online]. Available at: http://www.globefish.org/the-fishinfonetwork.html

Fishermen and Scientists Research Society (FSRS): FSRS is a non-profit organization to establish and maintain a network of fishermen and scientific personnel that are concerned with the long-term sustainability of the marine fishing industry in the Atlantic Region. The partnership facilitates collaborative research and the collection of relevant information that promotes the conservation of North Atlantic fisheries stocks. Source: [Online]. Available at: http://www.fsrs.ns.ca/

Indian Ocean and South-East Asian (IOSEA) Marine Turtle Memorandum of Understanding: The IOSEA Marine Turtle Memorandum of Understanding is an intergovernmental agreement that aims to protect, conserve, replenish and recover marine turtles and their habitats of the Indian Ocean and South-East Asian region, working in partnership with other relevant actors and organizations. Source: [Online]. Available at: http://ioseaturtles.org/

Institute of Marine Research (IMR): IMR provides research and management advice to ensure that Norway's marine resources are harvested in a sustainable way. Source: [Online]. Available at: http://www.imr.no

International Collective in Support of Fishworkers (ICSF): ICSF is an international non-governmental organization that works towards the establishment of equitable, gender-just, self-reliant and sustainable fisheries, particularly in the small-scale, artisanal sector. ICSF disseminates information on the issues of life, livelihood and living conditions of fishworkers around the world by maintaining a digital resource on legal instruments relevant to fisheries and fishing communities at http://legal.icsf.net/icsflegal/home.jsp.Source: [Online]. Available at: http://www.icsf.net/

International Council for the Exploration of the Sea (ICES): ICES is a multidisciplinary scientific forum for the exchange of information and ideas on all aspects of marine sciences pertaining to the North Atlantic, including the adjacent Baltic Sea and North Sea, and for the promotion and coordination of marine research within its member nations. Its principal functions are (1) to promote and coordinate marine research; (2) to publish and otherwise disseminate results of research; and (3) to provide scientific advice to member nation governments and international regulatory commissions. Source: [Online]. Available at: http://www.ices.dk/

International Institute of Fisheries Economics and Trade (IIFET): IIFET is an international group of economists, government managers, private industry members, and others interested in the exchange of research and information on marine resource issues. Their site at http://www.oregonstate.edu/dept/iifet/ is explorable for any aspect of fisheries, aquaculture, or marine resource economics, domestic or international trade in seafood, use of marine resources, fisheries management, publications and links to related Internet sites. Source: [Online]. Available at: http://oregonstate.edu/dept/

National Oceanic and Atmospheric Administration (NOAA) : NOAA is a federal agency focused on the condition of the oceans and the atmosphere. NOAA is dedicated to protecting and preserving the nation's living marine resources through scientific research, fisheries management, enforcement and habitat conservation. NOAA is a source of information on marine resources, ocean habitats and ecosystems. Source: [Online]. Available at: http://www.noaa.gov

Network of Aquaculture Centre in Asia Pacific (NACA): NACA is an intergovernmental organization that promotes rural development through sustainable aquaculture. NACA seeks to improve rural income, increase food production and foreign exchange earnings and to diversify farm production. The ultimate beneficiaries of NACA activities are farmers and rural communities. NACA supports institutional strengthening, technical exchange and the development of policies for sustainable aquaculture and aquatic resource management. Source: [Online]. Available at: http://www.enaca.org/

Network of Aquaculture Centres in Central-Eastern Europe (NACEE): NACEE is a voluntary association of Central and Eastern European aquaculture institutions. The main mandate of this network is to facilitate the research and development sphere in Central-Eastern Europe to be an integral part of the European Research Area. Source: [Online]. Available at: http://www.agrowebcee.net/nacee/about-nacee

South East Asian Fisheries Development Centre SEAFDEC: SEAFDEC is an autonomous inter-governmental body comprising of 11 Member Countries: Brunei Darussalam, Cambodia, Indonesia, Japan, Lao PDR, Malaysia, Myanmar, Philippines, Singapore, Thailand, and Vietnam. The Center operates through the Secretariat located in Thailand and four Technical Departments. SEAFDEC work to develop and manage the fisheries potential of the region by rational utilization of the resources for providing food security and safety to the people and alleviating poverty through transfer of new technologies, research and information dissemination activities. Source: [Online]. Available at: http://www.seafdec.org

United Nations Environment Programme(UNEP): UNEP is an international institution that coordinates United Nation's environmental activities, assisting developing countries in implementing environmentally sound policies and practices. Its activities cover a wide range of issues regarding the atmosphere, marine and terrestrial ecosystems, environmental governance and green economy. Source: [Online]. Available at: http://www.unep.org

World Aquaculture Society (WAS): WAS provides leadership for enhanced international communications, collaboration and information exchange as the progressive development and expansion of aquaculture is dependent on the generation, dissemination, and adoption of knowledge and technology. Source: [Online]. Available at: http://www.was.org

World Fish Centre (WFC): WorldFish, a member of the CGIAR Consortium, is an international, nonprofit research organization. CGIAR is a global partnership that unites organizations engaged in research for a food secure future. WorldFish works towards improving the livelihoods of those who are especially poor and vulnerable in places where fisheries and aquaculture can make a difference and, achieving large scale, environmentally sustainable, increases in supply and access to fish at affordable prices for poor consumers in developing countries. The research focuses on generating and synthesizing knowledge for sharing and helping to apply. Source: [Online]. Available at: http://www.worldfishcenter.org

Appendix 6 (Refer to Chapters 4 and 10)

International Fisheries Information Services and Products

Aquatic Commons: The Aquatic Commons is a thematic digital repository (http://aquacomm.fcla.edu/) covering the natural, marine, estuarine/brackish and freshwater environments. It includes all aspects of the science, technology, management and conservation of these environments, their organisms and resources, and the economic, sociological and legal aspects. The thematic digital repository is sponsored by the IAMSLIC and FAO has supported the development from its conception. It is complementary to OceanDocs., which is supported by the Intergovernmental Oceanographic Commission (IOC) specifically to collect, preserve and facilitate access to all research output from members of their Ocean Data and Information Network (ODINS). The records of both repositories are harvested by Avano which aggregates records from marine and aquatic repositories around the World. The repository aims to improve and facilitate the sharing of information on fisheries and aquaculture management. Source: [Online]. Available at: http://aquaticcommons.org/

Aquatic Sciences and Fisheries Abstracts (ASFA): Aquatic Sciences and Fisheries Abstracts (ASFA) is an abstracting and indexing service covering the world's literature on the science, technology, management, and conservation of marine, brackish water, and freshwater resources and environments, including their socio-economic and legal aspects. ASFA created in 1980 as an information partnership network that developed standards in the field of fisheries bibliographic references, together with the collection and collation of bibliographic references into the Global ASFA database. Source: [Online]. Available at: http://www.fao.org/fishery/asfa/en

Avano : Avano was a Marine and aquatic sciences OAI harvester of IAMSLIC. It offered access to more than 2 lakhs electronic resources about the marine and aquatic sciences-aquaculture and fisheries for instance but also geosciences, biology, ecology etc. These resources available in Avano came from the OAI harvesting of 289 Open Archives. This project was part of the Open Access International movement, which aimed at making scientific documentation accessible to a broad public through free publishing on the Web. French Research Institute for exploitation of the Sea (IFREMER) the hoisting agency (http://www.ifremer.fr/avano/)has closed the service with declining usage and limited staff available for support. Source: Retirement of Avano [Online]. Available at: http://www.iamslic.org

BIOSIS Zoological Record Plus (ZR Plus): ZR Plus, produced by Thomson Scientific, and formerly by BIOSIS and the Zoological Society of London, provides extensive coverage of the world's zoological articles and science literature, covering all research from biochemistry to veterinary medicine. Zoological Record produced by Thomson Reuters (Ovid interface) contains over 2 million bibliographic records with abstracts. Biosis Preview of Thomson Reuters combines journal content from Biological Abstracts with supplemental, non-journal coverage from Biological Abstracts /RRM (Reports, Reviews, Meetings) Source: [Online]. Serviced by: http://www.proquest.com/products-services/

CAB Abstracts: CAB Abstracts is the most comprehensive database covering international issues in agriculture, forestry, and allied disciplines in the life sciences. The database contains over 7 million bibliographic records from over 9,000 journals. Customers should seek an alternative supplier for their CABI subscription products. Source: CAB Products. [Online]. Available at: http://www.cabi.org/publishing-products/online-information-resources/cab-abstracts/

CODEX Alimentarius: Safe and sanitary processing of fishery products requires knowledge of acceptable and appropriate practices. Finding information on current best practices and government standards is critical. The CODEX Alimentarius develops food standards, guidelines and related texts such as codes of practice, specifically the Codex Committee on Fish and Fishery Products. Source: [Online] Available at: http://www.codexalimentarius.net / web/index_en.jsp) develops

Coordinating Working Party on Fisheries Statistics (CWP): The Coordinating Working Party on Fishery Statistics (CWP) provides a mechanism to coordinate fishery statistical programmes of regional fishery bodies and other inter-governmental organizations with a remit for fishery statistics of all marine water bodies. The FAO serves as the CWP Secretariat. Source: [Online]. Available at: http://www.fao.org/fishery/cwp/en

Directory of Open Access Journal: **DOAJ** provides access to over 3000 peer-reviewed journals that are freely available. DOAJ included nine numbers of fisheries journals in 2011. However, 52 journals in zoology and 24 in gender studies are also relevant and indicate the general breadth of coverage. Source: [Online]. Available at: https://doaj.org/

FAO Globefish is the unit in the FAO Fisheries and Aquaculture Department responsible for information on international fish trade. The core of GLOBEFISH is the GLOBEFISH Databank. GLOBEFISH produces a number of publications including fish price reports (European Fish Price Report), market studies (GLOBEFISH Research Programme) and trend analysis (GLOBEFISH Highlights). GLOBEFISH is jointly financed by FAO and GLOBEFISH Partners. GLOBEFISH is an integral part of the FISHINFO Network and performs a coordinating role in the Network activities. The information service covers a broad area, from the scientific and technical information required by the processing industry to market trends and prices, as well as the ever more complex requirements of international trade. Source: [Online]. Available at: http://www.globefish.org/

FAOLEX : FAO maintains a freely accessible database, FAOLEX (http://faolex.fao.org/faolex/) which has a global scope and links to the full text of national legislation relating to food, agriculture and renewable natural resources, including fisheries. Users of FAOLEX have direct access to the abstracts and indexing information about each text, as well as to the full text of most legislation contained in the database. Source: [Online]. Available at: http://faolex.fao.org

FishBase: FishBase is a relational database with information on fishes to cater to different professionals such as research scientists, fisheries managers, zoologists and many more. FishBase is the largest and most extensively accessed online database on adult finfish on the web. It has evolved into a dynamic and versatile ecological tool widely cited in scholarly publications. FishBase provides comprehensive species data, including information on taxonomy, geographical distribution, biometrics and morphology, behaviour and habitats, ecology and population dynamics as well as reproductive, metabolic and genetic data. Access to tools such as identification keys, biogeographical modeling, fishery statistics etc and direct species level links to information in other databases such as LarvalBase, GenBank, the IUCN Red List and the Catalog of Fishes are the features of FishBase. Source: [Online]. Available at: http://www.fishbase.org/

Fishery Resources Monitoring System (FIRMS): The Fisheries Resources Monitoring System (FIRMS) is a partnership of intergovernmental fisheries organizations that share a wide range of high-quality information on the global monitoring and management of marine fishery resources. The primary aim of the FIRMS is to provide access to a wide range of high-quality information on the global monitoring and management of fishery marine resources. FIRMS is part of the Fisheries Global Information System (FIGIS). Information provided by the partners is organized in a database and published in the form of fact sheets. Source: [Online]. Available at: http:// firms.fao.org/ firms/en

Fisheries Global Information System (FIGIS) is an information management tool that interconnects groups of institutional partnerships to build up a network of subsystems. FIGIS, as part of the FAO Fisheries and Aquaculture Department's regular activities acts as a framework with reference to FAO information management policy. FIGIS delivers expert knowledge, a set of software tools, collaborative mechanisms, and interoperability solutions to a broad range of needs in fisheries information. Source: [Online] Available at: http://www.fao.org/fishery/figis/en

Fish, Fisheries & Aquatic Biodiversity Worldwide Includes Twelve of the World's Major Fish and Fisheries Databases, such as: FISHLIT Aquatic Biology Citations (ABC), Fishing Industry Research Index (FIRI), Fisheries Review. This collection combines databases on all facets of ichthyology, fisheries, aquaculture, and aquatic & marine biology. Included in this remarkable resource are records from the now ceased database *Aquatic Biology, Aquaculture, & Fisheries Resources* (ABAFR), plus twelve of the world's major fish and fisheries databases. With excellent world coverage, this database includes research on aquaculture species ranging from culture and propagation to genetics, behavior, ecology and habitat. With nearly 1.5 million citations and abstracts dating back to the 1970s, this resource is essential for those dealing with all aspects of fish and aquatic biology. Source: [Online]. Serviced by https://www.ebscohost.com/academic/fish-fisheries-aquatic-biodiversity-worldwide

Food Science and Technology Abstracts (FSTA): FSTA is produced by the International Food Information Service (IFIS Publishing). It is the largest food science, food technology and food related human nutrition abstracts. FSTA covers journal articles (approximately 80%), patents, theses, standards, legislation, books, reviews, and conference proceedings. Source: http://library.dialog.com/bluesheets/ html/bl0051.html

Google Scholar is a freely accessible web search engine that indexes the full-text or metadata of scholarly literature across an array of publishing formats and disciplines. It provides mechanism to find the scientific journal literature cost effectively, although coverage is predominantly English language, commercial journals and links to freely available articles are limited. Source: [Online]. http://www.scholar.google.com

Information System for the Promotion of Aquaculture in the Mediterranean (SIPAM): SIPAM has been conceived with the aim of contributing to the Mediterranean aquaculture development through improving the flow of aquaculture information among the participating countries in the Mediterranean Basin. SIPAM was conceived in the early nineties on the observed fact that aquaculture cannot move forward without backing of an information system. SIPAM was an important step when 'informatics' level was poor and when an advanced information management system was absent. Source: [Online]. http://www.faosipam.org/

Ocean Biogeographic Information System (OBIS): Web-based provider of global geo-referenced information on marine species. OBIS allows users to search marine species datasets from all of the world's oceans and identify biodiversity hotspots and large-scale ecological patterns, analyze dispersions of species over time and space, and plot species locations with temperature, salinity and depth. Source: [Online]. http://www.iobis.org

Oceanic Abstracts: Oceanic Abstracts is focused exclusively on worldwide technical literature pertaining to the marine and brackish-water environment. The database focuses on living biology and physical oceanography, fisheries, aquaculture, non-living resources, meteorology, geology, plus environmental, technological, and legislative topics. Source: [Online]. Serviced by http://www.search.proquest.com/oceanic

OneFish: OneFish is a fishery projects portal and participatory resource gateway for the fisheries and aquatic research and development sector. It also hosts the Fish Technology Knowledge Base that facilitates networking for fish technologists It is possible for organizations and individuals to export to the Knowledge Base records (single, multiple or database) in a suitable format making it easier to up-date the Knowledge Base, encourage expansion of the network of contributors, and enhance the information available to users. The TorLib Fish Technology Database comprises more than 40,000 bibliographic references. OneFish is the most comprehensive and powerful resource gateway in the field of fisheries. OneFish is a Web based knowledge management system that draws together a broad cross section of stakeholders within the fisheries and aquatic research community. Source: [Online]. Available at: nopr.niscair.res.in/ bitstream/123456789/ 4681/1/ALIS% 2053(2)2096-102.pdf

Pacific Islands Marine Resources Information System (PIMRIS) : Pacific Islands Marine Portal of PIMRIS is a powerful resource gateway to Virtual Libraries and E-Repositories, Global Marine Databases and Resource Centres, Online Journals and information related to Pacific countries regarding country profiles, institutions, organizations, projects, Maps, GIS Data, training and educational resources etc. Source: [Online]. Available at: www.pimrisportal.org

Pollution Abstracts (PA): PA combines information on scientific research and government policies covering air pollution, marine pollution, freshwater pollution, sewage and wastewater treatment, waste management, land pollution, toxicology and health, noise, radiation and environmental action. Source: [Online]. Serviced by http://www.search.proquest.com/pollution

Regional Aquaculture Information System (RAIS)**:** RAIS groups all Member countries of the RECOFI Commission to facilitate the exchange of aquaculture information in the Gulf area and to develop an informal, flexible and functional network of regional experts to promote and develop the sector in the region. Source: [Online]. Available at: http://www.raisaquaculture.net/

United Nations Atlas of the Oceans: The UN Atlas of the Oceans is an Internet portal providing information relevant to the sustainable development of the oceans. It is designed for policy-makers who need to become familiar with ocean issues and for scientists, students and resource managers who need access to databases and approaches to sustainability. The UN Atlas can also provide the ocean industry and stakeholders with pertinent information on ocean matters. Source: [Online]. Available at: http://www.oceansatlas.org

Water Resources Abstracts: WRA provides summaries of the world's technical and scientific literature on water-related topics covering the characteristics, conservation, control, pollution, treatments and management of water resources. Abstracts are drawn from journals, books, conference proceedings, and technical reports in the physical and life sciences, as well as from engineering, legal and government publications. This database complements the Aquatic Sciences and Fisheries Abstracts (ASFA) database with the coverage of the marine environment and biological materials. Source: [Online]. Serviced by http://www.search.proquest.com/watersources

Waters & Oceans Worldwide: WOW is an electronic information resource which is an aggregation of 20 bibliographic databases from around the world. It covers records from the now-ceased database Marine Oceanographic and Freshwater Resources (MOFR), world's major water resource databases such as WATERLIT, The Freshwater Biological Association Library Catalogue, The International Water Management Institute Database (IMWI), AQUAREF, ACQUIRE, Delft Hydro, etc and all publications including journal articles, research reports, conference proceedings, grey literature, monographs, theses and dissertations, books, websites, etc. Provides keyword indexing, article abstracts, direct links to full text, etc. Source: [Online]. Serviced by https://www.ebscohost.com/academic/waters-oceans-worldwide & http://www.nisc.co.za/products/27/databases/waters-and-oceans-worldwide-wow

❑❑❑

Index

□□□